Practical Guide to Patch Testing

Eustachio Nettis • Gianni Angelini
Editors

Practical Guide to Patch Testing

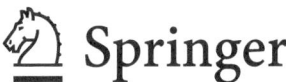 Springer

Editors
Eustachio Nettis
Allergist and Dermatologist
Regional Reference Center
University Allergology Clinic
Bari
Italy

Gianni Angelini
Professor of Dermatology
Former Professor and Chairman University
of Bari "Aldo Moro"
Bari
Italy

Partially based on the Italian language edition: Atlante e Compendio Il Patch Test, by E. Nettis and G. Angelini, Pacini-Editore Medicina, 2017. ©Pacini Editore

ISBN 978-3-030-33872-5   ISBN 978-3-030-33873-2   (eBook)
https://doi.org/10.1007/978-3-030-33873-2

© Springer Nature Switzerland AG 2020

This work is subject to copyright. All rights are reserved by the Publisher, whether the whole or part of the material is concerned, specifically the rights of translation, reprinting, reuse of illustrations, recitation, broadcasting, reproduction on microfilms or in any other physical way, and transmission or information storage and retrieval, electronic adaptation, computer software, or by similar or dissimilar methodology now known or hereafter developed.

The use of general descriptive names, registered names, trademarks, service marks, etc. in this publication does not imply, even in the absence of a specific statement, that such names are exempt from the relevant protective laws and regulations and therefore free for general use.

The publisher, the authors, and the editors are safe to assume that the advice and information in this book are believed to be true and accurate at the date of publication. Neither the publisher nor the authors or the editors give a warranty, expressed or implied, with respect to the material contained herein or for any errors or omissions that may have been made. The publisher remains neutral with regard to jurisdictional claims in published maps and institutional affiliations.

This Springer imprint is published by the registered company Springer Nature Switzerland AG
The registered company address is: Gewerbestrasse 11, 6330 Cham, Switzerland

Preface

Patch tests are the elective tests done to confirm the diagnosis of a contact dermatitis. They are essential tools in allergological practice. Even today, they are still the only method that can confirm or exclude the clinical suspicion of allergic contact dermatitis, and directly identify the etiological agent.

Over the years, the importance of patch tests has grown continually to such an extent that nowadays the results of these tests are also valid in the medicolegal field as allergological proof of an occupational disease.

Thus, it is extremely important to have an in-depth knowledge of the principles and practical rules governing the performance of these tests in order to obtain valid, reliable results and above all to offer the patient adequate guidance since the resolution of the disease and prevention of recurrence depend first and foremost on avoiding exposure to the substance responsible for the allergic manifestation.

This Atlas has the aim of providing specialists with a useful tool that can help them to gain experience of the correct methodology for performing patch tests. It offers an accurate information about the hapten series currently available (standard series and integrated series), their concentrations and correct preservation methods, as well as about the apparatus to be used to administer various tests. The vital aspects of reading and interpretation of the patch tests are closely analyzed, in view of the different clinical relevance of the possible reactions, in order to ensure the correct management of patients suffering from contact allergy.

Bari, Italy   Eustachio Nettis
                                                                            Gianni Angelini

Acknowledgment

Thanks for the irreplaceable collaboration to

Lucia Masciopinto, MD. Trainee Doctor in Allergology and Clinical Immunology

Stefania Magistà, MD. Trainee Doctor in Allergology and Clinical Immunology

Elisabetta Di Leo, MD, PhD. Specialist in Allergology and Clinical Immunology—PhD in Clinical Immunology

Maria Giovanna Priore, MD. Specialist in Allergology and Clinical Immunology

Contents

1. **Contact Dermatitis** 1
   Gianni Angelini and Eustachio Nettis

2. **Patch Testing** 5
   Eustachio Nettis, Domenico Bonamonte, and Gianni Angelini

3. **Reading of Patchtest Reactions** 21
   Eustachio Nettis, Caterina Foti, Daniele Paolo Pigatto,
   Alberico Motolese, and Gianni Angelini

4. **Evaluation of the Clinical Relevance of a Positive
   Patchtest Reaction** 33
   Eustachio Nettis and Gianni Angelini

5. **Management of the Allergic Patient** 41
   Gianni Angelini and Eustachio Nettis

6. **Other Techniques of Diagnosis** 43
   Gianni Angelini and Eustachio Nettis

7. **Examples of Patch Test Reactions and Related 72-h Readings** 45
   Gianni Angelini and Eustachio Nettis

Suggested Reading 71

Contributors

Gianni Angelini Dermatology, University of Bari "Aldo Moro", Bari, Italy

Domenico Bonamonte Department of Biomedical Science and Human Oncology, University of Bari "Aldo Moro", Bari, Italy

Caterina Foti Department of Biomedical Science and Human Oncology, University of Bari "Aldo Moro", Bari, Italy

Alberico Motolese Department of Dermatology, Macchi Hospital, Varese, Italy

Eustachio Nettis Department of Emergency and Organ Transplantation, University of Bari "Aldo Moro", Bari, Italy

Daniele Paolo Pigatto Department of Medical, Surgical and Dental Biosciences, Galeazzi Hospital, University of Milan, Milan, Italy

Contact Dermatitis

Gianni Angelini and Eustachio Nettis

As the shock-absorbing organ, the skin is the first line of defense against the various aggressive exogenous agents in the environment, including chemical substances. Interactions between the latter and the skin are often a cause of onset of contact dermatitis (CD), a multifactorial inflammatory complaint triggered by different pathogenic mechanisms and characterized by many different clinical-morphological pictures, as well as a variable evolution.

Among the various forms of eczema (exogenous and endogenous) (Table 1.1), CD is one of the most common clinical pictures and, indeed, one of the diseases most frequently observed in daily dermatological practice. The prevalence of CD in the general population ranges from 1.7% to 6.3% in the short term and from 6.2% to 10.6%, for longer-term disorders (1–3 years). The incidence of CD in the worker population accounts for 85–98% of all occupational skin disorders, which, in turn, occupy the first place among occupational diseases, or may follow immediately after musculoskeletal complaints and/or hearing damage, depending on the type of occupation.

Among the various clinical-pathogenic pictures of CD (Table 1.2), irritant contact dermatitis (ICD) is the one most commonly observed, especially in the occupational context. In fact, even a mild but chronic contact-induced irritation of the hands can affect nearly all subjects exposed to conditions in particular jobs, such as builders, hairdressers, fishermen and all those working with foodstuffs, as well as health-care staff, not to mention anyone doing housework.

G. Angelini
Dermatology, University of Bari "Aldo Moro", Bari, Italy
e-mail: gianniang@alice.it

E. Nettis (✉)
Department of Emergency and Organ Transplantation, University of Bari "Aldo Moro", Bari, Italy
e-mail: ambulatorio.allergologia@uniba.it

© Springer Nature Switzerland AG 2020
E. Nettis, G. Angelini (eds.), *Practical Guide to Patch Testing*,
https://doi.org/10.1007/978-3-030-33873-2_1

Table 1.1 Classification of types of eczema

Endogenous eczema
Atopic dermatitis
Seborrheic dermatitis
Nummular (discoid) eczema (also exogenous)
Pompholyx (dyshidrotic eczema) (also exogenous)
Asteatotic eczema (or hiemalis or craquelé)
Stasis eczema
Exogenous eczema
Irritant contact dermatitis
Allergic contact dermatitis
Microbial eczema

Table 1.2 Clinical forms of contact dermatitis

Irritant contact dermatitis
Allergic contact dermatitis
Irritant photocontact dermatitis
Allergic photocontact dermatitis
Airborne irritant contact dermatitis
Airborne allergic contact dermatitis
Non-eczematous contact dermatitis
Systemic contact dermatitis
Contact urticaria
Protein contact dermatitis

The interval between the harmful contact and the onset of CD (induction time) is not known because it depends on various exogenous environmental factors and endogenous human factors. In any case it is highly variable, ranging from hours or days (ICD due to strongly acidic or alkaline agents) to months or years (ICD due to toxic damage accumulating over time).

The different clinical appearances observed in the context of CD are attributable to factors such as the type of contact, chemical characteristics of the causal agents, and pathogenic mechanism involved. The point of evolution of the disease also contributes to the clinical-morphological variety of the disease, depending on whether it is observed during the acute, subacute, or chronic phase.

As regards the type of contact, a harmful chemical agent can reach the skin through two different routes, either exogenous or endogenous (Table 1.3). Exogenous contact can be "direct" (when a substance comes in direct contact with the skin, this being the most common form) or "airborne" (when it is diffuse in the environment and transported through the air, thereby coming in contact with the skin). This second type of exogenous contact occurs mainly in occupational fields. Direct and airborne exogenous contact can frequently occur together. Endogenous contact occurs in subjects whose skin is already sensitized, when they come in contact with substances that, besides acting topically, can also be administered systemically (drugs, foods, metals). There are various endogenous routes through which the allergen can reach the circulation system (Table 1.3).

Table 1.3 Types of skin contact

Exogenous route	
	Direct contact
	Airborne contact
Endogenous route	
	Oral
	Intravenous
	Intramuscular
	Rectal
	Inhalation
	Vesical
	Reconstructive surgery

1.1 Irritant Contact Dermatitis

This form of dermatitis is a non-immunological, toxic inflammatory reaction to external agents, prevalently of chemical type (irritants); important co-factors such as physical (mechanical, thermal, climatic) noxae also play a role, as well as endogenous factors. Among the latter, atopic dermatitis, previous or in course, is a risk factor for ICD of the hands in those who do wet work; furthermore, the dry skin of atopic subjects is itself very easily subject to irritant actions.

The innumerable irritant chemical agents present in the environment exert their harmful action through various different mechanisms, also depending on the substances present. They interfere with the different epidermic and dermic structures, activating all the cellular and chemical mediators of inflammation.

From the clinical standpoint, depending on the resistance of the various exposure sites and the intensity of action of the agent in question, an ample spectrum of lesions can be observed, ranging from simple dry skin through erythema, edema, vesico-bullous lesions, and desquamation up to necrosis. ICD can affect any skin site, generally remaining confined to the site of contact. In general, all subjects exposed to the harmful agent show some skin alterations, but of variable severity. The prognosis is normally good, featuring a fairly rapid damage repair response within a few days.

1.2 Allergic Contact Dermatitis

Allergic contact dermatitis (ACD) is a disease of both occupational and non-occupational concern; it develops due to a delayed-type cell-mediated sensitization following contact with various chemical substances.

The subjective symptoms of ACD are characterized by variable degrees of pruritus and objective symptoms by lesions that differ according to the disease phases: erythematous-edematous-vesicular areas with blurred margins in the acute phase; crusty, desquamative lesions with small dandruff strips in the subacute phase; and infiltrative lesions in the chronic phase.

Apart from the above classic eczematous clinical picture, ACD can manifest with non-classically eczematous pictures (polymorphous-like contact dermatitis, purpuric contact dermatitis, lichenoid contact dermatitis, lymphomatoid contact dermatitis, dyschromic contact dermatitis). Apart from sites of direct contact, ACD can present with clinical lesions at a distance from the primary focus. A possible severe complication, nowadays very rarely observed, is spread of the eczema to the entire skin (erythroderma). Although the complaint is subject to recurrence, the prognosis of ACD is good.

The diagnosis of ACD is based on two criteria, namely, the clinical findings and medical history and allergological aspects. The latter rely on various skin tests that include patch tests and photopatch tests.

Patch Testing

2

Eustachio Nettis, Domenico Bonamonte, and Gianni Angelini

2.1 Indications

Patch tests are *in vivo* diagnostic tests indicated if there is a suspicion of contact allergy, in order to identify the allergen responsible. They are also indicated in other dermatitis forms that could include secondary allergy to various haptens, or in some forms of adverse reactions to drugs.

To ensure their diagnostic efficiency, their administration must be entrusted to qualified, experienced specialists. The selection of the allergens to be tested in each patient is a fundamental part of the process, together with the correct preparation and application of the patch tests and their subsequent removal. Finally, the correct reading and interpretation of the results are of the utmost importance.

Patch tests are administered with the aid of a system consisting of the test apparatus and the hapten materials.

E. Nettis (✉)
Department of Emergency and Organ Transplantation, University of Bari "Aldo Moro", Bari, Italy
e-mail: ambulatorio.allergologia@uniba.it

D. Bonamonte
Department of Biomedical Science and Human Oncology, University of Bari "Aldo Moro", Bari, Italy
e-mail: domenico.bonamonte@uniba.it

G. Angelini
Dermatology, University of Bari "Aldo Moro", Bari, Italy
e-mail: gianniang@alice.it

2.2 Test Apparatus

The apparatus for patch tests includes the following:

1. A support (patch) used to position the hapten materials
2. A plaster attaching the support to the patient's skin

The plaster must guarantee adequate adhesion of the support and must be hypoallergenic (Scanpor®, Micropore®).

The test apparatus most commonly used in clinical practice includes the following: Al-test®, IQ Chamber®, and IQ Ultra®; Curatest F®; Finn and Large Chambers on Scanpor®; Van der Bend Square® and Haye's Test Chamber®.

In children the IQ Ultra® or Finn Chambers on Scanpor® are to be preferred owing to the smaller space on their backs (Figs. 2.1, 2.2, 2.3 and 2.4).

The test apparatus may already be mounted on a hypoallergenic plaster (e.g., Scanpor®, Micropore®). Nevertheless, to ensure adequate adhesion to the skin, in some cases it is best to add another hypoallergenic plaster (e.g., Eurofix® or Scanpor®) applied directly on the patient's back (Figs. 2.5, 2.6, 2.7, 2.8, 2.9, 2.10, 2.11, 2.12 and 2.13). The plasters can in rare cases be the cause of irritant or allergic reactions (Fig. 2.6).

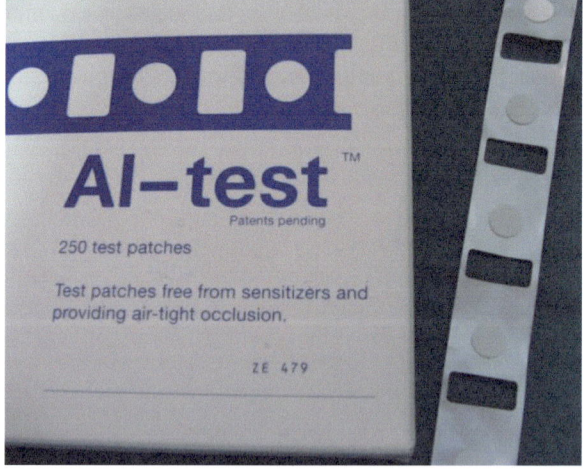

Fig. 2.1 Test apparatus: Al-test®

Fig. 2.2 Test apparatus: IQ Chamber®

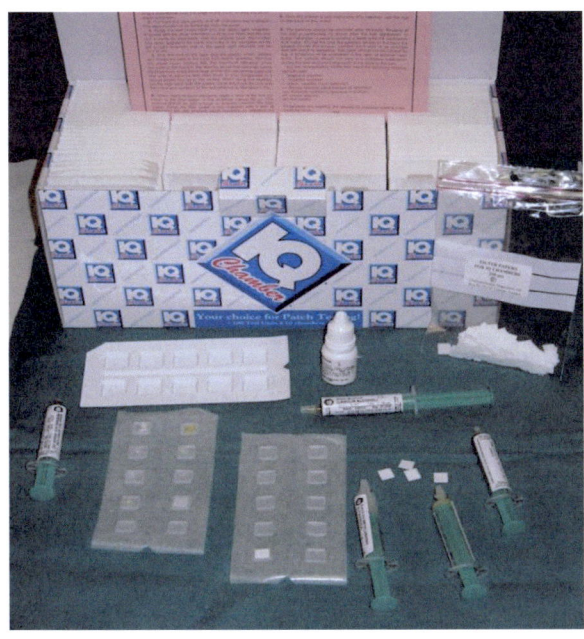

Fig. 2.3 Test apparatus: Finn Chamber®

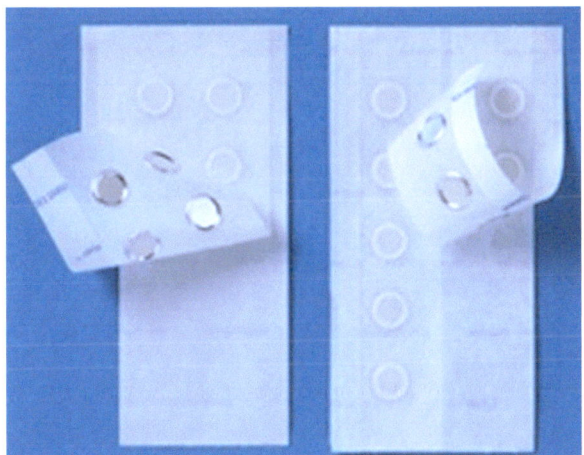

Fig. 2.4 Test apparatus: IQ Ultra®

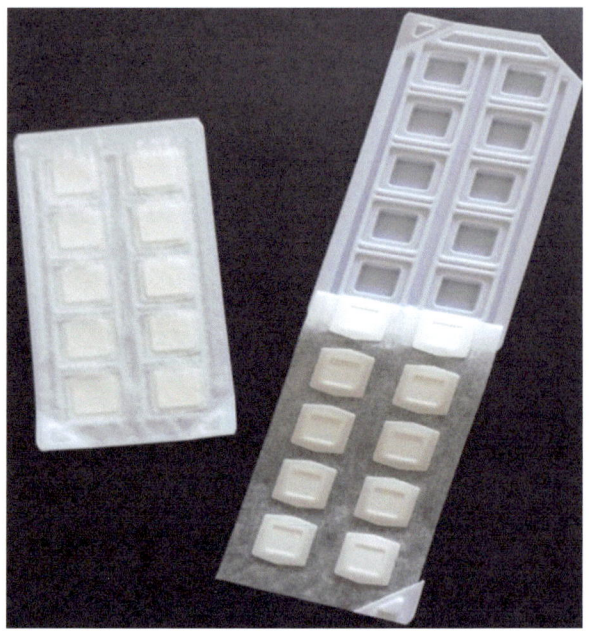

Fig. 2.5 Hypoallergenic plaster: Eurofix®

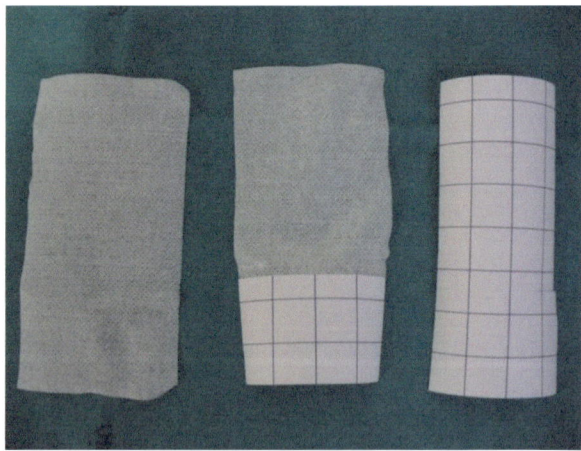

2 Patch Testing

Fig. 2.6 Skin reaction to adhesive plaster

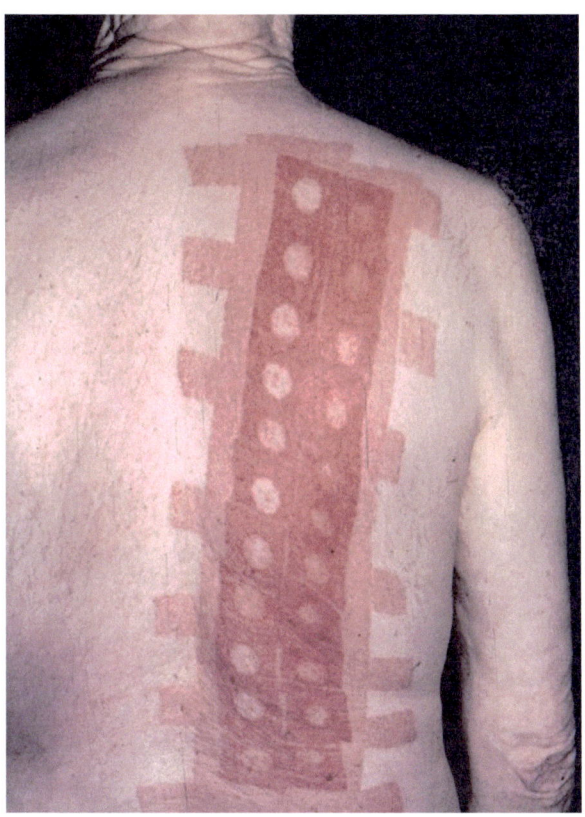

Fig. 2.7 Haptens in polypropylene syringes

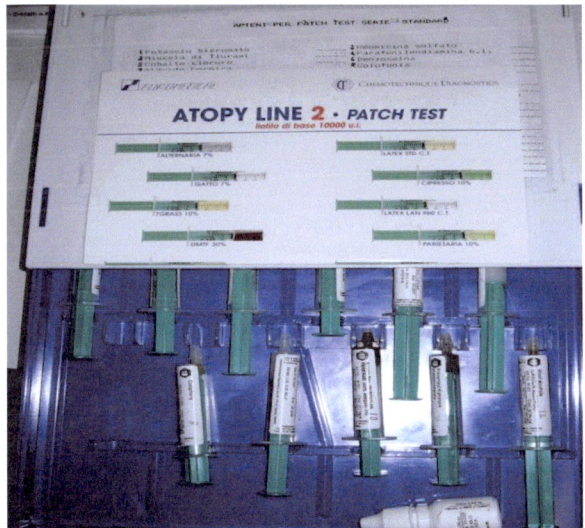

Fig. 2.8 Haptens in plastic vials

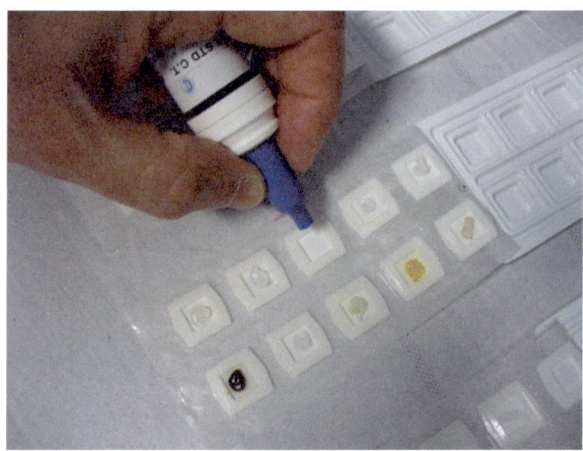

Fig. 2.9 Ready-to-use rapid tests: Expanded Standard series

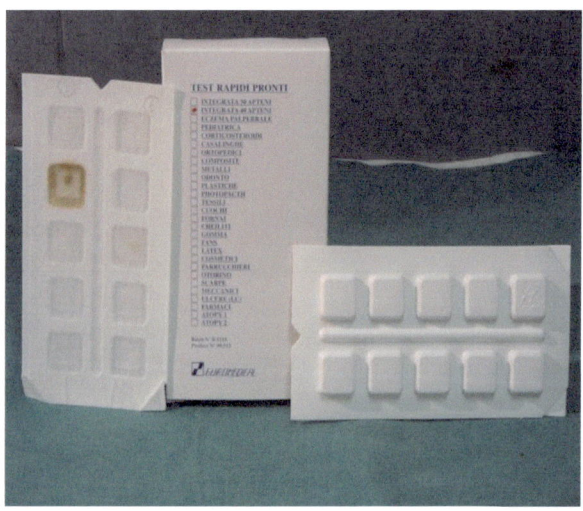

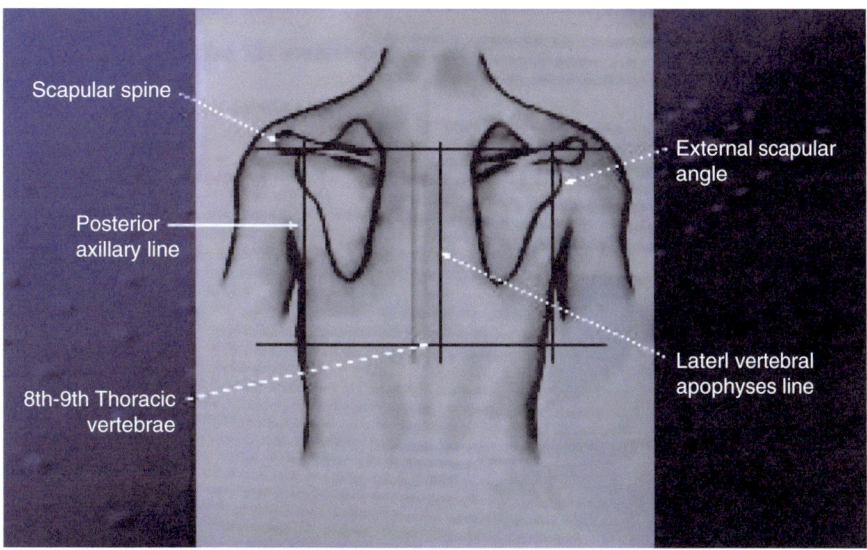

Fig. 2.10 Skin areas for the application of patch tests

Fig. 2.11 Application of a patch test

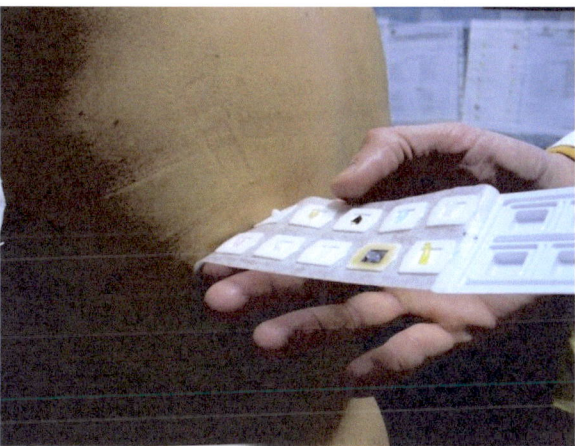

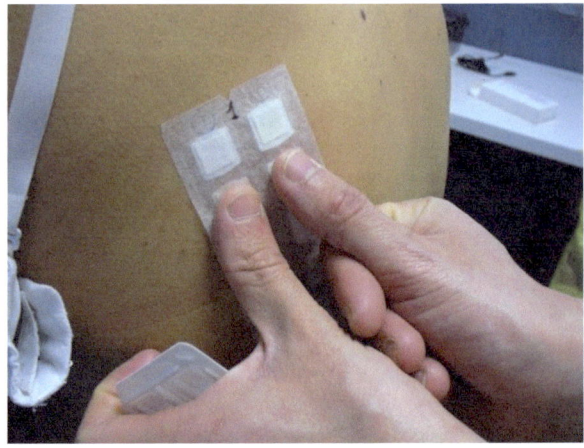

Fig. 2.12 Application of a patch test

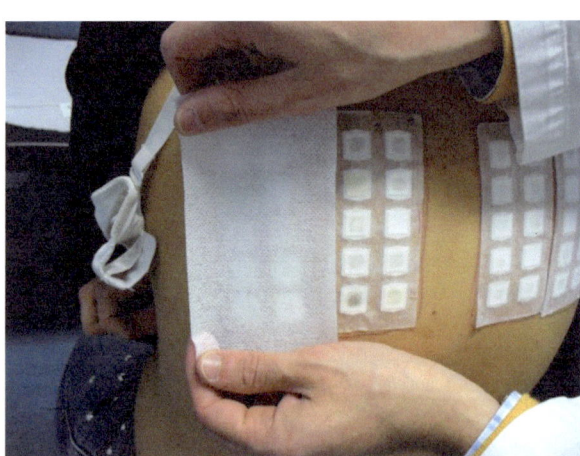

Fig. 2.13 Application of a patch test

2.3 Hapten Materials

Not all the substances with an allergenic potential are available for use as hapten materials.

Haptens are supplied by various companies. The same hapten materials are used in children as in adults. The patient is generally tested with a series of allergens including the most common haptens (main or standard series). The standard series in each nation consists of haptens whose allergenic incidence exceeds 1% (Table 2.1). In addition, depending on the clinical history, the site of the dermatitis, and in particular, the occupational risk or not, some haptens are added (integrated standard series), or other prescribed series of haptens (additional series), available on the market or directly prescribed by the physician.

Table 2.1 The most common allergens of a screening patch test series

Hapten	Concentration (vehicle)
Benzocaine	5%(pet)
Budesonide	0.01%(pet)
***p*-Tert-Butylphenolformaldehyde resin**	1%(pet)
Cobalt chloride	1%(pet)
Colophony	20%(pet)
Dimethylaminopropylamine	1%(aq)
Epoxy resin	1%(pet)
Formaldehyde	2%(aq)
Fragrance mix I	8%(pet)
Cinnamyl alcohol 1% Cinnamal 1% Hydroxycitronellal 1% Amyl cinnamal 1% Geraniol 1% Eugenol 1% Isoeugenol 1% Oakmoss absolute 1%	
Fragrance mix II	14%(pet)
Hexyl cinnamic aldehyde 5% Hydroxyisohexyl 3-cyclohexene carboxaldehyde 2.5% Farnesol 2.5% Coumarin 2.5% Citral 1% Citronellol 0.5%	
2-Hydroxyethyl methacrylate	2%(pet)
Imidazolidinyl urea	2%(aq)
***N*-Isopropyl-*N*′-phenyl-4-phenylenediamine (IPPD)**	0.1%(pet)
Lyral	5%(pet)
Mercapto mix	2%(pet)
2-(4-Morpholinylmercapto)benzothiazole (MOR) 0.5% Dibenzothiazyl disulfide (MBTS) 0.5% *N*-Cyclohexyl-2-benzothiazylsulfenamide 0.5% 2-Mercaptobenzothiazole (MBT) 0.5%	
2-Mercaptobenzothiazole	2%(pet)
Methylisothiazolinone + methylchloroisothiazolinone	0.02%(aq)
Neomycin sulfate	20%(pet)
Nickel sulfate	5%(pet)
Paraben mix	16%(pet)
Butylparaben 4.0% Ethylparaben 4.0% Methylparaben 4.0% Propylparaben 4.0%	
Peru balsam	25%(pet)
***p*-Phenylenediamine**	1%(pet)
Potassium dichromate	0.5%(pet)
Quaternium-15	1%(pet)
Textile dye mix	6.6%(pet)

(continued)

Table 2.1 (continued)

Hapten	Concentration (vehicle)
Disperse blue 35 (1%) Disperse yellow 3 (1%) Disperse orange 1 (1%) Disperse orange 3 (1%) Disperse red 1 (1%) Disperse red 17 (1%) Disperse blue 106 (0,3%) Disperse blue 124 (0,3%)	
Thimerosal	1% (pet)
Thiuram mix	1%(pet)
Dipentamethylenethiuram disulfide 0.25% Tetraethylthiuram disulfide 0.25% Tetramethylthiuram disulfide 0.25% Tetramethylthiuram monosulfide 0.25%	
Wool alcohols	30%(pet)

Table 2.2 shows a list of haptens that can be added to the standard series depending on the patient's clinical history of occupational or leisure exposure (standard series integrated according to the clinical history).

Table 2.3 shows one of the additional series used in clinical practice, together with the respective haptens.

Apart from the preconstituted haptens available on the market, other substances proposed and provided by the patient (extemporaneous preparations) can be tested. This may include some material as is (fabrics, plasters, rubbers, leather, cosmetics, plastics, fragrances, drugs for topical use), whereas most such substances (e.g., shampoo, hair perm substances, toothpastes) must be used at suitable concentrations after adding suitable vehicles or excipients (e.g., buffer solutions, vaseline). In these cases the patch test may be preceded by the administration of an open test or a semiopen test.

Generally, the allergenic creams available on the market are contained in polypropylene syringes (Fig. 2.7), and solutions in plastic vials with a dropper (Fig. 2.8).

The quantity of solid hapten material to be spread on the support is generally a filament measuring about 4–5 mm or a sufficient quantity to cover a little more than half the support surface. For liquids, one drop is sufficient for each hapten. Haptens must be kept refrigerated in the dark (8°–10°), except for wool alcohols, which must be kept at room temperature to prevent them from hardening. As to the sequence of haptens to be administered, it is advisable to avoid applying close together haptens that provoke intense reactions or cross-reactions, to reduce the risk of onset of an "excited skin syndrome." It is very important to make a careful selection of the allergens to be tested in each patient, employing the standard series and the integrated series, depending on the patient's clinical history, as well as the additional series.

Table 2.2 Haptens that can be added to the standard series

Hapten	Concentration (vehicle)
Diallyl disulfide	1% (pet)
Benzoyl peroxide	1% (pet)
Carba mix	3% (pet)
Wood tar mix	12% (pet)
Coal tar	5% (pet)
Quinoline mix	6% (pet)
N-(Cyclohexylthio)phthalimide	1% (pet)
Chlorhexidine digluconate	0.5% (aq)
Composite mix	5% (pet)
4-4-Diaminodiphenylmethane	0.5% (pet)
Ethylenediamine dihydrochloride	1% (pet)
Phenyl mercuric acetate	0.01% (aq)
Gentamicin sulfate	20% (pet)
Propylene glycol	5% (pet)
Imidazolidinyl urea	2% (pet)
Ketoprofen	1% (pet)
Latex LAN 960 C	100%
Sesquiterpene lactone mix	0.1% (pet)
Mercury(II)amidochloride	1% (pet)
Turpentine oil oxidized	0.4% (pet)
4-Aminoazobenzene	0.25% (pet)
2-Methoxy-6-n-pentyl-4-benzoquinone	0.01% (pet)
Promethazine hydrochloride	1% (pet)
Turpentine peroxide mix	0.4% (pet)

Table 2.3 Integrative textile series

Hapten	Concentration (vehicle)
Disperse blue 3	1% (vas)
Disperse blue 35	1% (vas)
Disperse blue 85	1% (vas)
Disperse blue 124	1% (vas)
Disperse blue 153	1% (vas)
Disperse brown 1	1% (vas)
Disperse orange 1	1% (vas)
Disperse orange 3	1% (vas)
Disperse red 1	1% (vas)
Disperse red 17	1% (vas)
Disperse yellow 3	1% (vas)
Disperse yellow 9	1% (vas)
Melamine formaldehyde	7% (vas)
Ethylene urea	1% (vas)
Urea formaldehyde resin	10% (vas)
Dimethylol dihydroxy ethylene urea	4.5% (aq)

2.4 Rapid Tests

Some test apparatus systems include both the support containing the allergen material and the plaster. The advantages of rapid tests (Fig. 2.9) can be summarized as a combination of their rapid execution and ease of transport and hence the possibility of use in less central outpatient clinics. The disadvantages are their higher costs compared to the traditional method and the risk that the method may be administered by non-expert operators.

2.5 Photopatch Tests

Photopatch tests are used in order to diagnose allergic contact photodermatitis. Table 2.4 shows the series of the most common photohaptens. However, depending on the clinical history, other substances considered possible culprits of the photodermatitis can be tested, if necessary together with others with a chemical affinity, to reveal any cross-reactions. Photohaptens must be exposed to UVA rays. The most commonly used light sources are fluorescent lamps with a low mercury pressure:

Table 2.4 Common photoallergens

Hapten	Concentration (vehicle)
Butylmetoxydibenzoylmethane	5% (pet)
Homosalate	5% (pet)
3-4-Methylbenylon camphor	10% (pet)
Benzophenone-3	10% (pet)
Octyl mytoxycinnamate	2% (pet)
Phenylbenzimidazol-5-sulfonic acid	2% (pet)
Benzophenone-4	2% (pet)
Drometizole trisiloxane	10% (pet)
Octocrylene	10% (pet)
Octylsalicilate	10% (pet)
Isoamyl-*p*-methoxycinnamate	1% (pet.)
Terephtalydene dicamphor sulphonic acid (mexoryl sx)	1% (pet)
Bis ethylhexyloxyphenol methoxyphenyl triazine	1% (pet)
Methylene bis benzotriazolyl tetramethylbutylphenol	1% (pet)
2-(4 Diethylamino-2 hydroxybenzoil) benzoic acid hexyl ester	1% (pet)
Disodium phenyldibenzimidazone tetrasulphonate	1% (pet)
Diethylhexyl butamidotriazone	1% (pet)
Polysilicone 15	1% (pet)
Ketoprofen	1% (pet)
Etofenamate	10% (pet)
Piroxicam	1% (pet)
Diclofenac sodium salt	1% (pet)
Ibuprofen	1% (pet)

three "blacklight" types at 320–450 nm and three "sunlamp" types at 280–340 nm positioned in a glass-covered booth to eliminate the UVB rays. The UVA dosages to be employed range from 1 to 10 J/cm^2, depending on the phototype (generally 5 J/cm^2, placing the lamp 25 cm away from the patient's back). Photopatch test substances are applied in dual order as parallel series on each side of the back. One of the two series is removed after 24 h and the uncovered skin area is exposed to the ultraviolet rays. The results are read 24 h later, together with the other series, which have been regularly removed after 48 h. Further readings are made after 72–96 h from the test application. A photoallergic reaction is diagnosed only if it is present on the irradiated zone and absent on the contralateral non-irradiated zone. The result may be defined as a "combined" or "photo-aggravated" reaction if it is present on both sides, but at a greater intensity on the photoexposed site. The presence of positive reactions of the same intensity on both sides will suggest a simple contact allergy. The reading parameters, quali-quantitative assessments, and disadvantages of photopatch tests are the same as those reported above for patch tests.

2.6 Contraindications

Patch tests should not be administered if:

- There is acute or diffuse eczema, to avoid false-positive "excited skin syndrome" reactions or worsening of the dermatitis.
- The patient is undergoing systemic corticosteroid therapy or immunosuppressive drugs (it is necessary to wait for an interval consisting of the duration of the drug half-life multiplied by five before administering such a test), or even topical corticosteroid therapy on the area where the patch must be placed (wait for 7 days after the last administration), since these generally have a suppressant influence and so reduce the positivity of the test. In addition, a reduced intensity response will occur if the patient is receiving oral cyclosporin A.
- The patient is receiving oral cinnarizine or ketotifen.
- The environmental temperature or degree of humidity is high, because the test apparatus is more likely to detach.
- During pregnancy, even if fetal damage has never been demonstrated.
- The patient is exposed to UVB-UVA rays; in very tanned patients, the test should not be administered less than 4 weeks after the last exposure to the sun.

2.7 Application Method

To ensure a correct interpretation of the results, the appropriate patch test application technique must be applied. The supports must be applied on the upper back (the lower back, being less sensitive, can give rise to false-negative reactions), in a zone with no skin lesions nor hairs. For each hemithorax, it is better to choose the upper area bordered by lines that pass through the scapular spine, outside the posterior

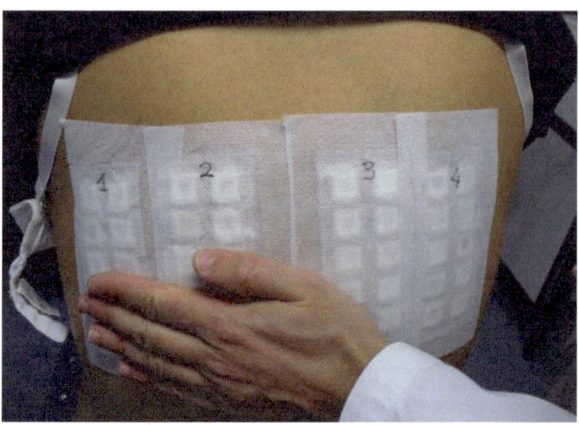

Fig. 2.14 Application of a patch test

axillary line, medially to the lateral vertebral apophyses, and the lower area running through the spinal apophyses of the eighth to ninth thoracic vertebrae (Fig. 2.10). If necessary, the zone can be shaved, preferably the day before the application, using an electric razor or a razor blade, refraining from applying shaving cream or soap. If the skin is oily, it is better to cleanse it with ethanol or another mild solvent. The test strips should be applied bottom-up. Light pressure is exerted to prevent mixing of the haptens. Each support will then be numbered using a felt-tip pen. Finally, light manual pressure is exerted on the plaster to ensure that it sticks to the skin, as well as making sure there is an adequate distribution of the haptens (Figs. 2.11, 2.12, 2.13 and 2.14). The supports must not be applied on pigmented moles or similar lesions, because if they were to become irritated, they could complicate the test readings. In situations where application of the plaster on the patient's back is impossible (e.g., in cases of diffuse acne), the external face of the arm can be used, or the anterior surface of the thigh.

2.8   Patient's Information

During the patch test application sessions, the patient should be given some verbal and/or written recommendations concerning the correct norms to be complied with (Table 2.5).

2.9   Removal

The test apparatus is removed 48 h after application. Generally during removal, the sites where each allergen was placed, and the external margins of the patch, are marked on the skin (Fig. 2.15). A fluorescent ink pen, which is practically invisible

2 Patch Testing

Table 2.5 Information for the patient scheduled to undergo patch testing

Do not bathe or shower
Do not make abrupt movements that could detach the patches
Try to avoid sweating
Avoid excessive physical effort
Avoid sun exposure
Do not scratch even if you feel itching
Re-attach any patch if it detaches from the skin using a sticking plaster
Remember that the test may induce worsening of the dermatitis
Go immediately to the outpatient clinic, even the day after the test, if intense local or general reactions develop

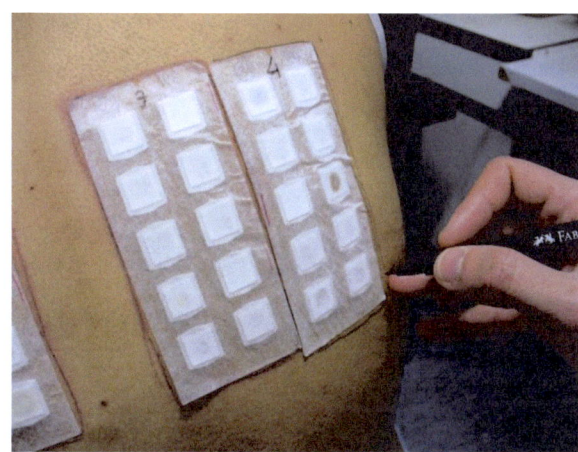

Fig. 2.15 Removal of the patch test

to the naked eye, can be used for this purpose. When the patient returns to the outpatients clinic for the next reading, under the Wood lamp ultraviolet rays, the ink may highlight the reactions. This method is esthetically acceptable to the patient and causes less damage to clothing than a common felt-tip pen. After the removal of the test apparatus, to better outline the contact area of each hapten, a rectangular Euromedical® Caliber can be used, of the same size as the patches (Fig. 2.16). The first reading is made 30–60 min after removal of the patch. A second reading is made at 72 h (1 day after removal of the patches) or 96 h (2 days after removal). Finally, a last reading can be made at 1 week after the application of the patches. The main reason why readings are done at variable times after removal of the patches is that there is a high percentage of delayed positive reactions in areas that appeared negative or doubtful at the time of removal 48 h after application of the tests. The substances most likely to elicit this type of reactions are nickel, lanolin, paraphenylenediamine, neomycin, cobalt, gold, and chromium. Moreover, comparing the results of late readings with the early results can help to differentiate an

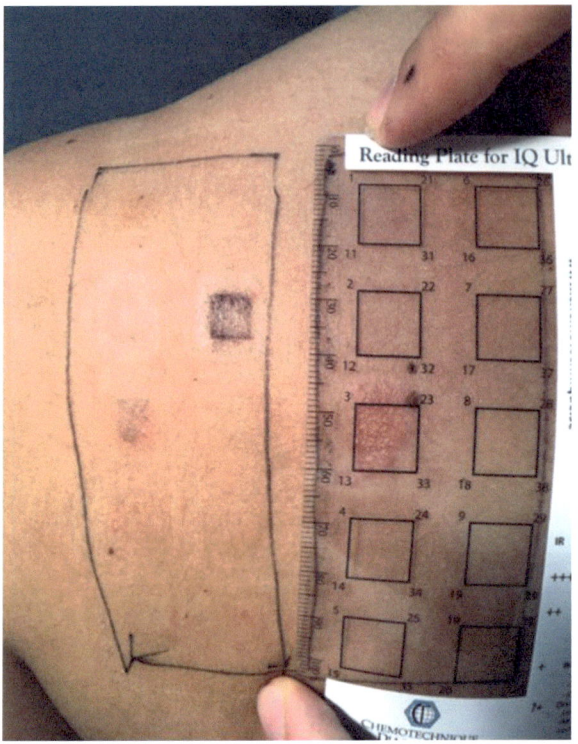

Fig. 2.16 Rectangular caliber

irritant-type reaction (that will be evident at 48 h and will regress within 1–2 days) from an allergic reaction (evident after 48–72 h and longer lasting, taking a long time to regress). It is clear that even if patients may regard a reading after 7 days as inconvenient, they will readily understand the advantages of an accurate and complete evaluation of the results. Nevertheless, some specialists remove the apparatus after 72 h and make a single reading 30–60 min after the removal, inviting the patient to go to the outpatient clinic once more if a delayed reaction should develop.

Reading of Patchtest Reactions

3

Eustachio Nettis, Caterina Foti, Daniele Paolo Pigatto, Alberico Motolese, and Gianni Angelini

A scrupulous evaluation of the reactions must be made by using a magnifying glass, carrying out digital palpation, and assessing symptoms. Delayed reactions to patch tests can be positive, false positive, false negative, doubtful, and mixed (Table 3.1).

Table 3.1 Delayed reactions to patch tests

Positive reactions
False-positive reactions
False-negative reactions
Doubtful reactions
Mixed reactions

E. Nettis (✉)
Department of Emergency and Organ Transplantation, University of Bari "Aldo Moro", Bari, Italy
e-mail: ambulatorio.allergologia@uniba.it

C. Foti
Department of Biomedical Science and Human Oncology, University of Bari "Aldo Moro", Bari, Italy
e-mail: caterina.foti@uniba.it

D. P. Pigatto
Department of Medical, Surgical and Dental Biosciences, Galeazzi Hospital, University of Milan, Milan, Italy
e-mail: paolo.pigatto@unimi.it

A. Motolese
Department of Dermatology, Macchi Hospital, Varese, Italy
e-mail: alberico.motolese@ospedale.varese.it

G. Angelini
Dermatology, University of Bari "Aldo Moro", Bari, Italy
e-mail: gianniang@alice.it

3.1 Positive Reactions

After making a qualitative-quantitative assessment, positive reactions are classified according to the criteria listed in Table 3.2.

Positive reactions, meaning specific allergy results, must be differentiated from false-positive results. Table 3.3 shows the differential criteria for distinguishing positive from false-positive results. When differentiating these reactions, note must be taken not only of the symptoms evoked by the reaction but also of the margins, structure, and shape of the reaction.

Table 3.2 Qualitative-quantitative assessment of allergic reactions (Figs. 3.1, 3.2, 3.3, and 3.4)

Doubtful +?	Weak erythema
Mild +	Uniform erythema with edema (raised skin appreciable at palpation), possible papules or slight blistering
Strong++	Erythema, edema (skin appreciable at palpation), evident papules and/or vesicles that may extend beyond the application area
Intense+++	Erythema, edema, very evident papules and vesicles, which are sometimes confluent, forming bullae
IR	Irritant reaction with a different morphology
NT	Not tested

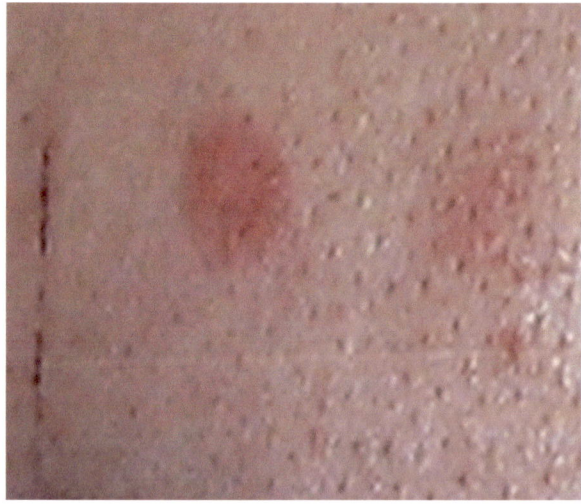

Fig. 3.1 Weak erythema: +? (doubtful reaction)

3 Reading of Patchtest Reactions

Fig. 3.2 Uniform erythema with edema, some papules or a hint of vesicles+

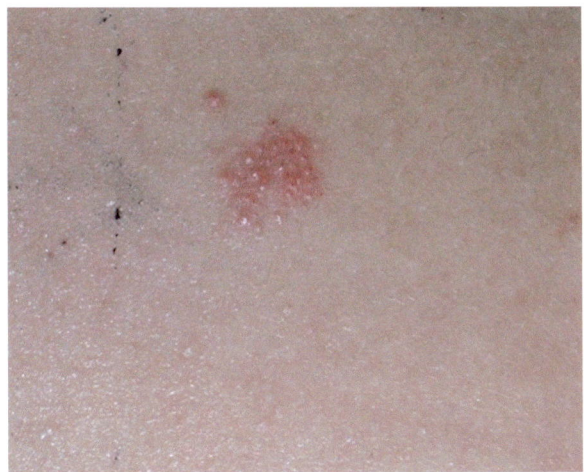

Fig. 3.3 Erythema, edema, evident papules and/or vesicles extending beyond the test area: ++

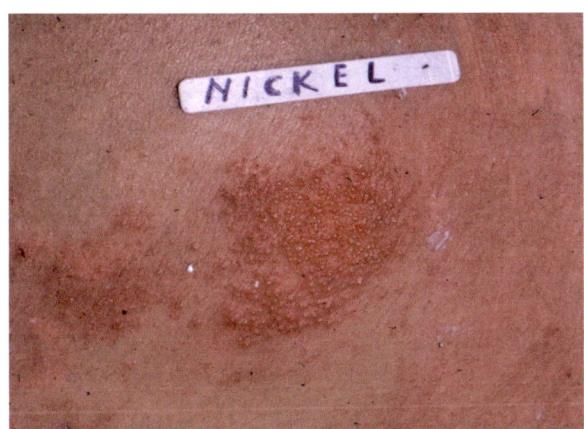

Fig. 3.4 Erythema, edema, very evident papules and vesicles, sometimes confluent forming blisters: +++

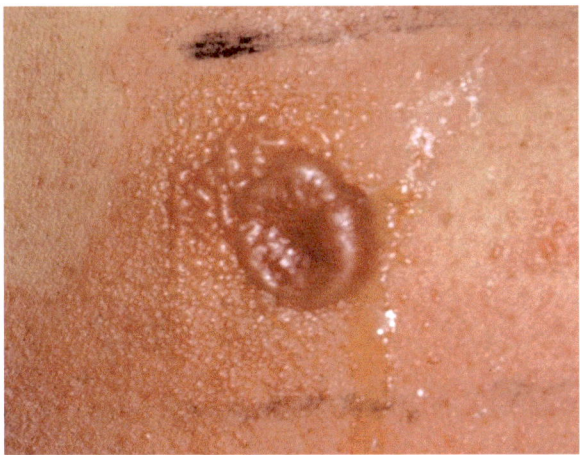

Table 3.3 Criteria employed to differentiate positive reactions from false-positive reactions

	Positive reaction, allergy	False-positive reaction, irritant type
Time of onset	After 48–72 h or more	After a few hours
Evolution	Increasing intensity after removal of the test apparatus	Regression after removal of the test apparatus
Symptoms	Pruritus	Burning or pricking sensation
Morphology	Erythema, edema, vesicles, sometimes confluent forming bullae Skin thickening at palpation	Brown erythema, papules and pustules, vesicles (rare), blisters. No skin thickening at palpation
Reaction margins	Irregular and blurred, extending beyond the hapten contact area	Distinct, coinciding with the hapten contact area
Structure	Homogeneous: the lesions are homogeneously distributed on the contact area	Nonhomogeneous: dyshomogeneous distribution of the lesions on the reaction area
New acute dermatitis presentation	Possible	No
Test with the same concentrations	Negative in controls	Positive in controls

Table 3.4 False-positive reactions

Erythematous reactions
Erythematous-purpuric reactions
"Chapping reactions" or "soap" or "shampoo" effects
"Glazed reactions"
"Margin effect"
Pustulous reaction
Papulous follicular reaction
Blistering reaction
Necrotic reaction
Eczematous reaction due to "excited skin syndrome"
Reactions due to other skin diseases, new or preexistent

3.2 False-Positive Reactions

False-positive reactions manifest with different pictures (Table 3.4). The most common causes are shown in Table 3.5.

Erythematous reaction. An erythematous reaction is generally considered false positive when it has a nonhomogeneous distribution (see Sect. 3.5).

Erythematous-purpuric reaction. Generally caused by cobalt (Fig. 3.5).

"Chapping reaction" or "soap" or "shampoo" effect. These reactions have very clear-cut margins, with minor erythema, accentuation of the skin folds, and desquamation caused by haptens with a tensioactive power (quaternary ammonium salts, soaps, and shampoos) (Fig. 3.6).

3 Reading of Patchtest Reactions

Table 3.5 The most common causes of false-positive reactions

Too high a concentration of the hapten
Application of excessive antigen quantities
Irritant vehicle
Presence of impurities in the tested substance
Presence of eczematous lesions on the patch test application site
Execution of patch tests during the active disease phase
Highly irritable condition of the skin
Intense reaction to the plaster
Non-uniform blending of the test substance with the vehicle
Solid material pressure effect
"Excited skin syndrome" phenomenon

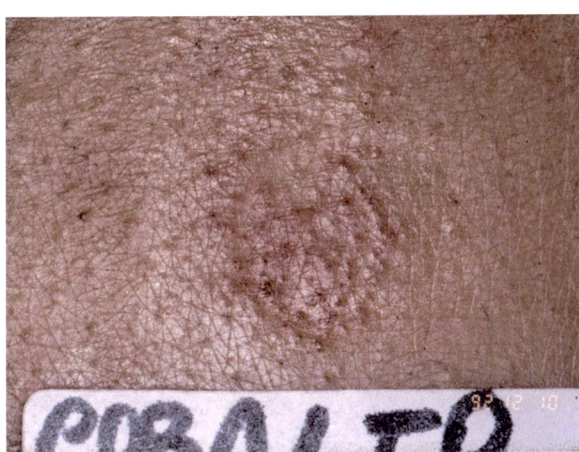

Fig. 3.5 False positive reaction: purpuric

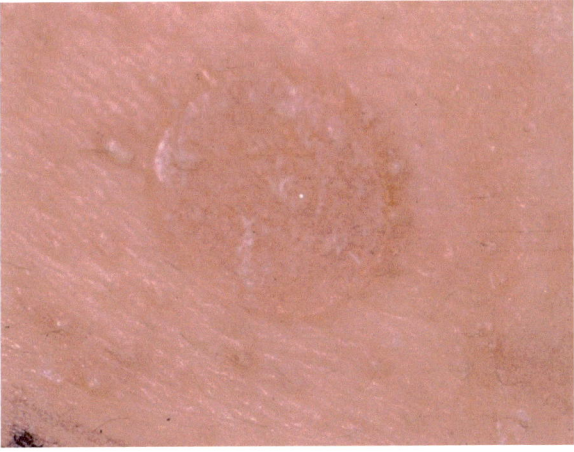

Fig. 3.6 False positive reaction: soap or shampoo effect

"Glazed reactions." The affected skin is shiny, brownish, and erythematous, with distinct margins; it shows microerosions and detaches if contrary pressure is applied.

"Margin effect." This occurs when the hapten material accumulates in a ring on the borders of the test area and acquires irritant properties. In such cases the reaction will appear as an erythematous ring. However, in some cases the reaction may be a positive allergic reaction, causing blisters (this occurs with allergens like corticosteroids or haptens in acetone) (Fig. 3.7).

Pustulous reactions. Characterized by the presence of skin pustules, sometimes with minor erythema and not pruriginous, localized at the follicular level but above all at the openings of the sweat glands. This is more common in children and atopic subjects and is generally caused by contact with metals (Fig. 3.8).

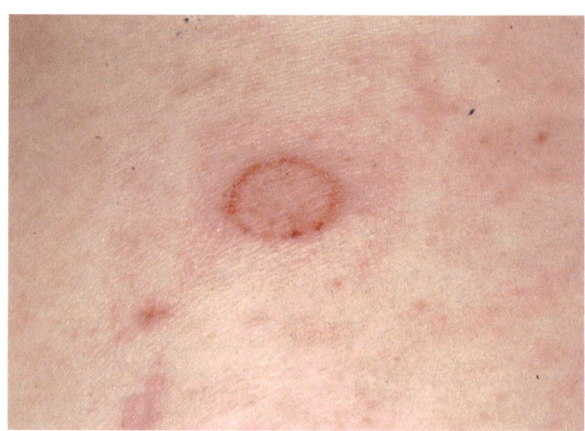

Fig. 3.7 False positive reaction: "margin effect"

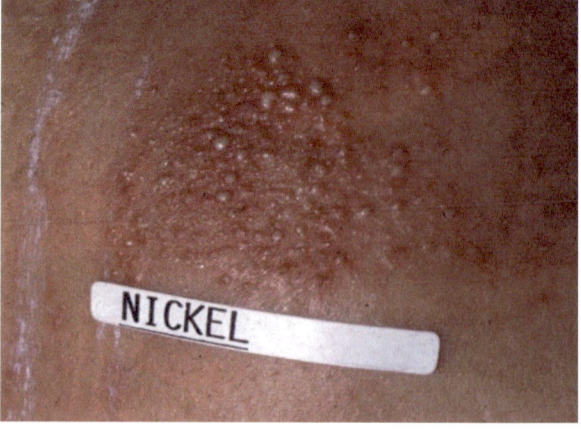

Fig. 3.8 False positive reaction: pustulous

Papulous follicular reactions. These are erythematous-papulous reactions, mostly at follicular sites, and are caused by poorly homogenized hapten materials (Fig. 3.9).

Bullous reactions. These can easily be mistaken for intense positive reactions, but there will be evident peripheral vesicles and pruritus. They are most commonly caused by contact with strong acids (Fig. 3.10).

Necrotic reactions. They are characterized by necrotic tissues and are due to very irritant substances (Fig. 3.11).

Eczematous "excited skin syndrome" reactions. See Sect. 3.6.

Isomorphic reactions due to supravening or preexistent skin diseases. These reactions show the typical morphology of the other supravening or preexistent skin diseases (lichen planus, psoriasis, acne, seborrheic dermatitis, miliaria crystallina or rubra disease) (Fig. 3.12).

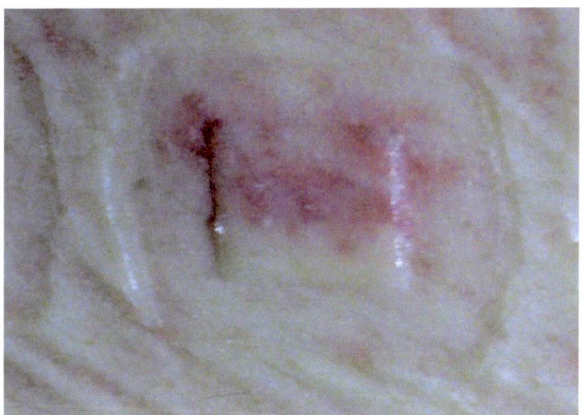

Fig. 3.9 False positive reaction: papulous, follicular

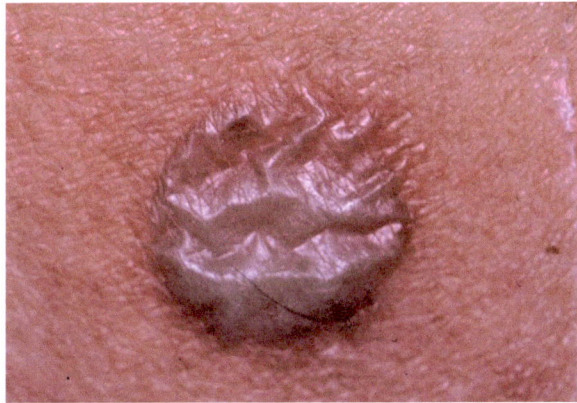

Fig. 3.10 False positive reaction: bullous

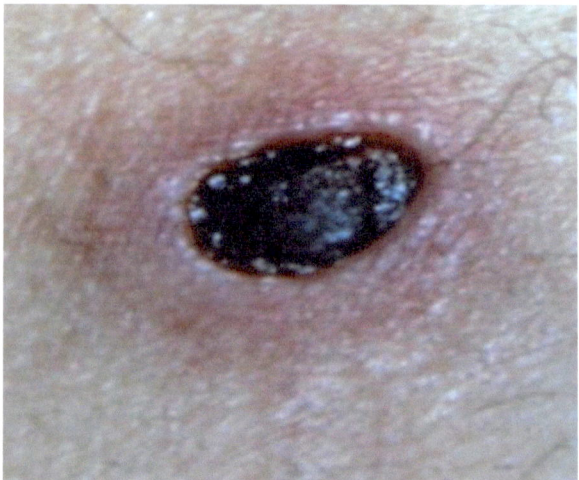

Fig. 3.11 False positive reaction: necrotic

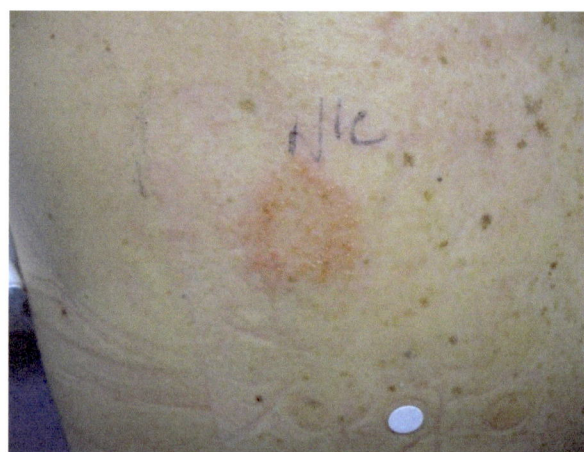

Fig. 3.12 False positive reaction: miliary crystaline

3.3 False-Negative Reactions

False-negative reactions are negative reactions to patch tests in patients suffering from contact allergy. They are mostly due to factors correlated to the hapten materials:

- Insufficient hapten concentration or quantity applied.
- The method employed: insufficient occlusion, partial detachment of the test apparatus caused by sweating, and too early a reading time.
- Failure to apply the test on the recommended site.
- Absence of the hapten responsible for the allergic contact dermatitis in the test series.
- The need to employ photopatch testing.
- Patient characteristics: a low sensitivity level below the test limit of detection and refractory disease following an acute eczema episode.

Fig. 3.13 Mixed reaction

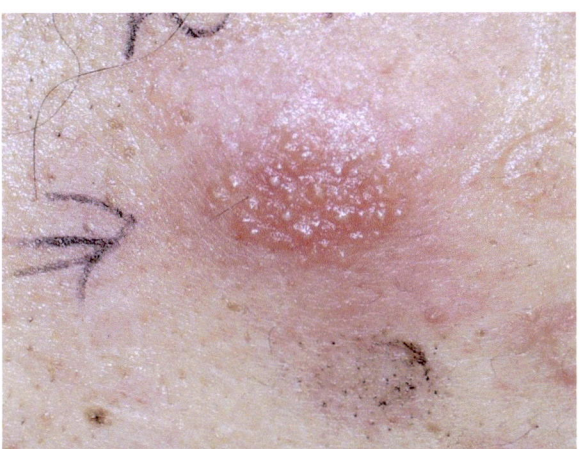

- Therapies in course: systemic corticosteroid or immunosuppressant treatments and local corticosteroid therapy on the test site.
- Exposure to UV rays.

In some of the above-reported cases, if false-negative reactions develop, the patch tests can be repeated after 7 days (when the first patch test will have increased the level of sensitivity), using the suspect hapten at a greater concentration and applying it to a more sensitive site (lateral face of the arm), or after removing the superficial skin sites by de-greasing the skin with ether, or skin stripping with adhesive tape, or else by scarification (applying a scratch-patch test).

3.4 Mixed Reactions

Mixed reactions are characterized by the coexistence of both allergic type components (e.g., vesicles) and irritant-type manifestations (e.g., pustules). In cases of a mixed response, the patch tests should be repeated (Fig. 3.13).

3.5 Doubtful Reactions

Doubtful reactions (+?) may consist of a nonhomogeneous or also only a homogeneous erythema (Figs. 3.14 and 3.15). It should be remembered that erythema is in any case a parameter indicating the degree of intensity, which does not allow an allergic-type reaction to be distinguished from an irritant type. In cases of doubtful reactions, characterized by erythema alone, the test must be repeated at a later time. In fact, when repeated, the doubtful reaction could manifest as a "positive allergic reaction." This occurs more frequently in cases of doubtful reactions characterized by a homogeneous erythema than by a nonhomogeneous reaction.

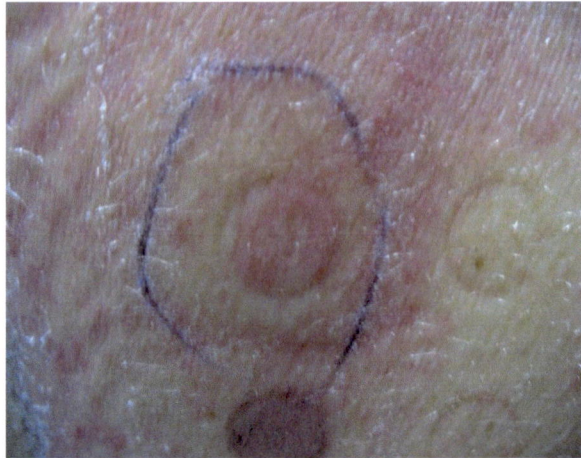

Fig. 3.14 Doubtful reaction: homogeneous erythema

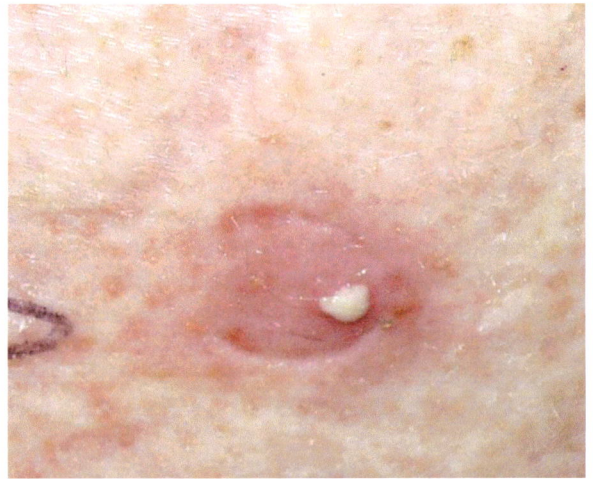

Fig. 3.15 Doubtful reaction: non homogeneous erythema

3.6 Side Effects

Some side effects and complications caused by patch tests are reported.

3.6.1 Active Sensitization (Spontaneous Flare-Up)

Active sensitization reactions appear as positive reactions after at least 7 days from the application of the test apparatus (generally around the 15th day). They are caused by the interaction of an allergen with the newly sensitized tissues. If another patch test is then applied with the same substance, the positive reaction will appear within 48–72 h. The most frequent cause of active sensitization is the use of allergenic materials at very high concentrations, these often not being standardized materials. This *ex novo* sensitization may regress if no further contact with the hapten occurs.

3.6.2 Reactions Due to Systemic Absorption of the Hapten

A new acute phase of the dermatitis: A positive patch test may also be accompanied by a new acute phase of the existing or preexisting dermatitis caused by the same allergen but in this case systemically absorbed.

Reactions at the level of other organs: This is an exceptional observation and may consist of bronchial asthma or angioedema; an anaphylactic reaction may even develop.

Such reactions are IgE-mediated, and the onset occurs a few minutes after the application of the patch test in sensitized patients.

3.6.3 "Excited Skin Syndrome"

"Excited skin syndrome," also known as "angry back," is a phenomenon attributable to skin hyper-reactivity. Above all, in cases of an intense positive reaction to a given substance, other possible positive reactions can develop, but these must in such circumstances be regarded as doubtful (Fig. 3.16). In fact, it has been demonstrated that about 40% of these apparently positive reactions are really false-positive reactions.

The hyper-reactivity phenomonen is not restricted to the back and could even involve the patient's whole skin. To reduce the risk of onset of this phenomenon, the dermatologist should avoid testing substances that can induce an intense reaction in

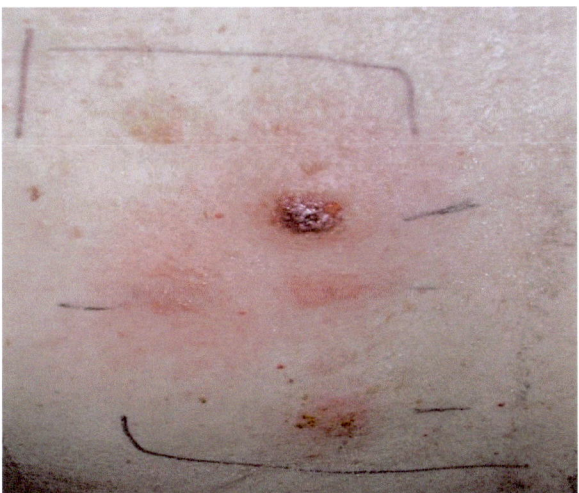

Fig. 3.16 "Excited skin syndrome"

nearby positions and also refrain from performing patch tests when the eczema is in an acute phase or spreading. A further useful precaution is the use of anallergic plasters.

In cases when several positive responses to patch tests are obtained, the medical history needs to be examined in greater depth to confirm whether these positive reactions have a true significance.

The dermatologist can proceed in two different ways:

- Retest the positive substances singly, one at a time at least 1 week apart, in particular if they are substances that are ubiquitous in the environment, or difficult to avoid, or if a medico-legal question is involved in terms of the allergen responsible.
- Avoid retesting the positive substances if the patient can easily avoid contact with them, or if the medical history fails to confirm any relevance.

Evaluation of the Clinical Relevance of a Positive Patchtest Reaction

Eustachio Nettis and Gianni Angelini

Positive reactions to patch tests must be carefully evaluated to judge their clinical relevance, in terms of any relation between the positive reaction and the patient's dermatitis. Such clinical relevance may be:

- Present (occupational and/or non-occupational): Related to the clinical symptoms that led the patient to seek dermatological attention (the patient has suffered exposure to the allergen that resulted positive to the test responsible for the current dermatitis).
- Past (occupational and/or non-occupational): Related to past clinical events, not directly correlated to those currently complained of (the patient was exposed in the past to the allergen that resulted positive to the test that had triggered a known previous dermatitis).
- Present+past (occupational and/or non-occupational): This situation is related to the allergic contact dermatitis that has long been in course and features a chronic-recurrent trend.
- Due to exposure: In this case there is a history of evident exposure to the allergen, but it is not responsible for the current or previous contact dermatitis (positive reaction to thimerosal).

E. Nettis (✉)
Department of Emergency and Organ Transplantation, University of Bari "Aldo Moro", Bari, Italy
e-mail: ambulatorio.allergologia@uniba.it

G. Angelini
Dermatology, University of Bari "Aldo Moro", Bari, Italy
e-mail: gianniang@alice.it

Table 4.1 Pitfalls in the assessment of clinical relevance

Contacts and data fail to emerge during medical history probing occupational aspects
Contacts and data fail to emerge during medical history probing leisure activities aspects
Hobbies during free time not assessed
Contacts with flowers, plants, and inhalant products not considered
Cosmetic products not mentioned
Medications and parapharmaceuticals not mentioned
Volatile substances in the environment (indoors and outdoors) in the form of powders, fumes, vapors, and gases not mentioned
Substances used by the patient (topical medications, cosmetics, hair dyes, condoms, clothing contaminated by substances at the workplace, etc.) not considered
Substances not patch-tested (but the standard series usually demonstrate up to about 70% of cases of allergy)
"Delayed" reactions not recorded (about 2% of positive reactions are observed after more than 72 h)
Patch testing with patient-supplied products not done
Impurities, e.g., in cosmetics, not assessed: Produced by containers, by chemical interactions, and by physical or chemical decomposition

- Unknown: This is related in some cases to a clinically latent sensitization to a given allergen, which becomes manifest after the application of the patch test, showing a positive reaction even if the patient has never previously had any form of dermatitis.

The assessment of clinical relevance of a positive patch test reaction is a complex process with many pitfalls (Table 4.1).

It is clear that to make a close evaluation of the clinical relevance of a positive reaction to a patch test, the clinical history must be very carefully analyzed and a thorough clinical examination made after reading the patch tests. The patch test response module must also contain a point reporting on the relevance of positive reactions (Tables 4.2, 4.3, 4.4, 4.5, and 4.6).

4 Evaluation of the Clinical Relevance of a Positive Patchtest Reaction

Table 4.2 Example of the patch test response form with positive (++) reaction to the hapten thiuram mix in patient with hands contact dermatitis, triggered and aggravated with the use of rubber gloves

Baseline Patch Test Series

Mr/Mrs_____Date_____

Benzocaine 5% (pet)	Mercapto mix 2% (pet) 2-(4-Morpholinylmercapto)benzothiazole (MOR) 0.5% Dibenzothiazyl disulfide (MBTS) 0.5% N-Cyclohexyl-2-benzothiazylsulfenamide 0.5% 2-Mercaptobenzothiazole (MBT) 0.5%
Budesonide 0.01% (pet)	2-Mercaptobenzothiazole 2% (pet)
p-Tert-Butylphenolformaldehyde resin 1% (pet)	Methylisothiazolinone+methylchloroisothiazolinone 0.02% (aq)
Cobalt chloride 1% (pet)	Neomycin sulfate 20% (pet)
Colophony 20% (pet)	Nickel sulfate 5% (pet)
Dimethylaminopropylamine 1% (aq)	Paraben mix 16% (pet) Butylparaben 4.0% Ethylparaben 4.0% Methylparaben 4.0% Propylparaben 4.0%
Epoxy resin 1% (pet)	Peru balsam 25% (pet)
Formaldehyde 2% (aq)	p-Phenylenediamine 1% (pet)
Fragrance mix I 8% (pet) Cinnamyl alcohol 1% Cinnamal 1% Hydroxycitronellal 1% Amyl cinnamal 1% Geraniol 1% Eugenol 1% Isoeugenol 1% Oakmoss absolute 1%	Potassium dichromate 0.5% (pet)
Fragrance mix II 14% (pet) Hexyl cinnamic aldehyde 5% Hydroxyisohexyl 3-cyclohexene carboxaldehyde 2.5% Farnesol 2.5% Coumarin 2.5 % Citral 1% Citronellol 0.5%	Quaternium -15 1% (pet)
2-Hydroxyethyl methacrylate 2% (pet)	Textile dye mix 6.6% (pet) Disperse blue 35 (1%) Disperse yellow 3 (1%) Disperse orange 1 (1%) Disperse orange 3 (1%) Disperse red 1 (1%) Disperse red 17 (1%) Disperse blue 106 (0,3%) Disperse blue 124 (0,3%)
Imidazolidinyl urea 2% (aq)	Thimerosal 1% (pet)
N-Isopropyl-N'-phenyl-4-phenylenediamine 0.1% (pet)	**Thiuram mix 1% (pet) ++** **Dipentamethylenethiuram disulfide 0.25%** **Tetraethylthiuram disulphide 0.25%** **Tetramethylthiuram disulphide 0.25%** **Tetramethylthiuram monosulphide 0.25%**
Lyral 5% (pet)	Wool alcohols

CONCLUSIONS   POSITIVE   [X]   NEGATIVE   [ ]

POSITIVITY_____ Thiuram mix _____ RELEVANCE _____ Present _____

The MD in charge

Table 4.3 Example of the patch test response form with positive (++) reaction to the hapten *p*-phenylenediamine base in a patient with fingers contact dermatitis, caused by detergent liquids. From the anamnesis emerges, however, the presence of previous eczematous scalp manifestations (not present now), arising after the use of a dark hair dye

Baseline Patch Test Series

Mr/Mrs_____ Date _____

Benzocaine 5% (pet)	Mercapto mix 2% (pet) 2-(4-Morpholinylmercapto)benzothiazole (MOR) 0.5% Dibenzothiazyl disulfide (MBTS) 0.5% N-Cyclohexyl-2-benzothiazylsulfenamide 0.5% 2-Mercaptobenzothiazole (MBT) 0.5%
Budesonide 0.01% (pet)	2-Mercaptobenzothiazole 2% (pet)
p-Tert-Butylphenolformaldehyde resin 1% (pet)	Methylisothiazolinone+methylchloroisothiazolinone 0.02% (aq)
Cobalt chloride 1% (pet)	Neomycin sulfate 20% (pet)
Colophony 20% (pet)	Nickel sulfate 5% (pet)
Dimethylaminopropylamine 1% (aq)	Paraben mix 16% (pet) Butylparaben 4.0% Ethylparaben 4.0% Methylparaben 4.0% Propylparaben 4.0%
Epoxy resin 1% (pet)	Peru balsam 25% (pet)
Formaldehyde 2% (aq)	*p*-Phenylenediamine 1% (pet) ++
Fragrance mix I 8% (pet) Cinnamyl alcohol 1% Cinnamal 1% Hydroxycitronellal 1% Amyl cinnamal 1% Geraniol 1% Eugenol 1% Isoeugenol 1% Oakmoss absolute 1%	Potassium dichromate 0.5% (pet)
Fragrance mix II 14% (pet) Hexyl cinnamic aldehyde 5% Hydroxyisohexyl 3-cyclohexene carboxaldehyde 2.5% Farnesol 2.5% Coumarin 2.5 % Citral 1% Citronellol 0.5%	Quaternium -15 1% (pet)
2-Hydroxyethyl methacrylate 2% (pet)	Textile dye mix 6.6% (pet) Disperse blue 35 (1%) Disperse yellow 3 (1%) Disperse orange 1 (1%) Disperse orange 3 (1%) Disperse red 1 (1%) Disperse red 17 (1%) Disperse blue 106 (0,3%) Disperse blue 124 (0,3%)
Imidazolidinyl urea 2% (aq)	Thimerosal 1% (pet)
N-Isopropyl-N'-phenyl-4-phenylenediamine 0.1% (pet)	Thiuram mix 1% (pet) Dipentamethylenethiuram disulfide 0.25% Tetraethylthiuram disulphide 0.25% Tetramethylthiuram disulphide 0.25% Tetramethylthiuram monosulphide 0.25%
Lyral 5% (pet)	Wool alcohols

CONCLUSIONS   POSITIVE   [X]   NEGATIVE   [ ]

POSITIVITY_____ *p*-Phenylenediamine(PPD) _____ RELEVANCE_____ Past_____

The MD in charge

4 Evaluation of the Clinical Relevance of a Positive Patchtest Reaction

Table 4.4 Example of patch test response form with positive (++) reaction to the hapten *p*-phenylenediamine base in a patient with scalp contact dermatitis, caused by a hair dye. The anamnesis shows the presence of previous eczematous clinical manifestations triggered always in the same places by the use of dyes

Baseline Patch Test Series

Mr/Mrs_____Date _____

Benzocaine 5% (pet)	Mercapto mix 2% (pet) 2-(4-Morpholinylmercapto)benzothiazole (MOR) 0.5% Dibenzothiazyl disulfide (MBTS) 0.5% N-Cyclohexyl-2-benzothiazylsulfenamide 0.5% 2-Mercaptobenzothiazole (MBT) 0.5%
Budesonide 0.01% (pet)	2-Mercaptobenzothiazole 2% (pet)
p-Tert-Butylphenolformaldehyde resin 1% (pet)	Methylisothiazolinone+methylchloroisothiazolinone 0.02% (aq)
Cobalt chloride 1% (pet)	Neomycin sulfate 20% (pet)
Colophony 20% (pet)	Nickel sulfate 5% (pet)
Dimethylaminopropylamine 1% (aq)	Paraben mix 16% (pet) Butylparaben 4.0% Ethylparaben 4.0% Methylparaben 4.0% Propylparaben 4.0%
Epoxy resin 1% (pet)	Peru balsam 25% (pet)
Formaldehyde 2% (aq)	*p*-Phenylenediamine 1% (pet) ++
Fragrance mix I 8% (pet) Cinnamyl alcohol 1% Cinnamal 1% Hydroxycitronellal 1% Amyl cinnamal 1% Geraniol 1% Eugenol 1% Isoeugenol 1% Oakmoss absolute 1%	Potassium dichromate 0.5% (pet)
Fragrance mix II 14% (pet) Hexyl cinnamic aldehyde 5% Hydroxyisohexyl 3-cyclohexene carboxaldehyde 2.5% Farnesol 2.5% Coumarin 2.5 % Citral 1% Citronellol 0.5%	Quaternium-15 1% (pet)
2-Hydroxyethyl methacrylate 2% (pet)	Textile dye mix 6.6% (pet) Disperse blue 35 (1%) Disperse yellow 3 (1%) Disperse orange 1 (1%) Disperse orange 3 (1%) Disperse red 1 (1%) Disperse red 17 (1%) Disperse blue 106 (0,3%) Disperse blue 124 (0,3%)
Imidazolidinyl urea 2% (aq)	Thimerosal 1% (pet)
N-Isopropyl-N'-phenyl-4-phenylenediamine 0.1% (pet)	Thiuram mix 1% (pet) Dipentamethylenethiuram disulfide 0.25% Tetraethylthiuram disulphide 0.25% Tetramethylthiuram disulphide 0.25% Tetramethylthiuram monosulphide 0.25%
Lyral 5% (pet)	Wool alcohols

CONCLUSIONS   POSITIVE   X   NEGATIVE ☐

POSITIVITY_____ *p*-Phenylenediamine(PPD) base_____RELEVANCE_____Present and Past____

The MD in charge

Table 4.5 Example of compilation of patch test response form with positive reaction (++) to thimerosal in a patient with contact dermatitis in the right wrist, caused by the watch strap. From the anamnesis emerges the use in the past of ophthalmic eye drops containing thimerosal

Baseline Patch Test Series

Mr/Mrs_____ Date _____

Benzocaine 5% (pet)	Mercapto mix 2% (pet) 2-(4-Morpholinylmercapto)benzothiazole (MOR) 0.5% Dibenzothiazyl disulfide (MBTS) 0.5% N-Cyclohexyl-2-benzothiazylsulfenamide 0.5% 2-Mercaptobenzothiazole (MBT) 0.5%
Budesonide 0.01% (pet)	2-Mercaptobenzothiazole 2% (pet)
p-Tert-Butylphenolformaldehyde resin 1% (pet)	Methylisothiazolinone+methylchloroisothiazolinone 0.02% (aq)
Cobalt chloride 1% (pet)	Neomycin sulfate 20% (pet)
Colophony 20% (pet)	Nickel sulfate 5% (pet)
Dimethylaminopropylamine 1% (aq)	Paraben mix 16% (pet) Butylparaben 4.0% Ethylparaben 4.0% Methylparaben 4.0% Propylparaben 4.0%
Epoxy resin 1% (pet)	Peru balsam 25% (pet)
Formaldehyde 2% (aq)	*p*-Phenylenediamine 1% (pet) ++
Fragrance mix I 8% (pet) Cinnamyl alcohol 1% Cinnamal 1% Hydroxycitronellal 1% Amyl cinnamal 1% Geraniol 1% Eugenol 1% Isoeugenol 1% Oakmoss absolute 1%	Potassium dichromate 0.5% (pet)
Fragrance mix II 14% (pet) Hexyl cinnamic aldehyde 5% Hydroxyisohexyl 3-cyclohexene carboxaldehyde 2.5% Farnesol 2.5% Coumarin 2.5 % Citral 1% Citronellol 0.5%	Quaternium-15 1% (pet)
2-Hydroxyethyl methacrylate 2% (pet)	Textile dye mix 6.6% (pet) Disperse blue 35 (1%) Disperse yellow 3 (1%) Disperse orange 1 (1%) Disperse orange 3 (1%) Disperse red 1 (1%) Disperse red 17 (1%) Disperse blue 106 (0,3%) Disperse blue 124 (0,3%)
Imidazolidinyl urea 2% (aq)	**Thimerosal 1% (pet) ++**
N-Isopropyl-N'-phenyl-4-phenylenediamine 0.1% (pet)	Thiuram mix 1% (pet) Dipentamethylenethiuram disulfide 0.25% Tetraethylthiuram disulphide 0.25% Tetramethylthiuram disulphide 0.25% Tetramethylthiuram monosulphide 0.25%
Lyral 5% (pet)	Wool alcohols

CONCLUSIONS   POSITIVE   [X]   NEGATIVE   [ ]

POSITIVITY_____ Thimerosal_____ RELEVANCE_____ Esposition____

The MD in charge

4 Evaluation of the Clinical Relevance of a Positive Patchtest Reaction

Table 4.6 Example of patch test response form with positive (++) reaction to the hapten neomycin sulfate in a patient with hands contact dermatitis, caused by the use of detergents. From the anamnesis, however, there is no dermatitis caused by topical products containing neomycin

Baseline PatchTest Series

Mr/Mrs_____ Date _____

Benzocaine 5% (pet)	Mercapto mix 2% (pet) 2-(4-Morpholinylmercapto)benzothiazole (MOR) 0.5% Dibenzothiazyl disulfide (MBTS) 0.5% N-Cyclohexyl-2-benzothiazylsulfenamide 0.5% 2-Mercaptobenzothiazole (MBT) 0.5%
Budesonide 0.01% (pet)	2-Mercaptobenzothiazole 2% (pet)
p-Tert-Butylphenolformaldehyde resin 1% (pet)	Methylisothiazolinone+methylchloroisothiazolinone 0.02% (aq)
Cobalt chloride 1% (pet)	**Neomycin sulfate 20% (pet) ++**
Colophony 20% (pet)	Nickel sulfate 5% (pet)
Dimethylaminopropylamine 1% (aq)	Paraben mix 16% (pet) Butylparaben 4.0% Ethylparaben 4.0% Methylparaben 4.0% Propylparaben 4.0%
Epoxy resin 1% (pet)	Peru balsam 25% (pet)
Formaldehyde 2% (aq)	p-Phenylenediamine 1% (pet) ++
Fragrance mix I 8% (pet) Cinnamyl alcohol 1% Cinnamal 1% Hydroxycitronellal 1% Amyl cinnamal 1% Geraniol 1% Eugenol 1% Isoeugenol 1% Oakmoss absolute 1%	Potassium dichromate 0.5% (pet)
Fragrance mix II 14% (pet) Hexyl cinnamic aldehyde 5% Hydroxyisohexyl 3-cyclohexene carboxaldehyde 2.5% Farnesol 2.5% Coumarin 2.5% Citral 1% Citronellol 0.5%	Quaternium-15 1% (pet)
2-Hydroxyethyl methacrylate 2% (pet)	Textile dye mix 6.6% (pet) Disperse blue 35 (1%) Disperse yellow 3 (1%) Disperse orange 1 (1%) Disperse orange 3 (1%) Disperse red 1 (1%) Disperse red 17 (1%) Disperse blue 106 (0,3%) Disperse blue 124 (0,3%)
Imidazolidinyl urea 2% (aq)	Thimerosal 1% (pet)
N-Isopropyl-N'-phenyl-4-phenylenediamine 0.1% (pet)	Thiuram mix 1% (pet) Dipentamethylenethiuram disulfide 0.25% Tetraethylthiuram disulfide 0.25% Tetramethylthiuram disulfide 0.25% Tetramethylthiuram monosulfide 0.25%
Lyral 5% (pet)	Wool alcohols

CONCLUSIONS   POSITIVE   [X]   NEGATIVE [   ]

POSITIVITY_____ Neomycin sulfate _____ RELEVANCE_____ Unknown _____

The MD in charge

Management of the Allergic Patient

Gianni Angelini and Eustachio Nettis

Subject to the evaluation of the clinical relevance of a positive patch test reaction, the expert will provide information to the patient, giving a general description of the culprit substance (what it is, where it may be found), advising on how to avoid contact with it and with others that may cause a cross-reaction with the allergen and which alternative substances can be used, if possible. Finally, the medical specialist will provide the patient with an information sheet, containing further, in depth information about the previously discussed substance (Table 5.1).

G. Angelini
Dermatology, University of Bari "Aldo Moro", Bari, Italy
e-mail: gianniang@alice.it

E. Nettis (✉)
Department of Emergency and Organ Transplantation, University of Bari "Aldo Moro", Bari, Italy
e-mail: ambulatorio.allergologia@uniba.it

Table 5.1 Example of "information card" for nickel allergic patients

Useful information for patients allergic to nickel
If the patch tests performed showed that **you are allergic to nickel**:
Can I recover from this allergy?
Certainly you can recover from the current dermatitis but further exposures to nickel could cause a recurrence and any contact must be therefore avoided. At the present time, it is not possible to undergo any form of "vaccination" to improve the patient's conditions or complete recovery from the disorder.
Hypersensitizing vaccination
It is possible to undergo hypersensitizing treatment, in highly intense nickel allergy cases, where the patient's quality of life is seriuosly affected. A specialist must prescribe the treatment, monitoring progresses. The treatment consists of ingesting capsules containing nickel, to be taken three times a week for 6 months
Where is nickel to be found?
A complete list of objects and products containing nickel would be very long, so here are mentioned few common items including:
– **Jewelry:** earrings (even those defined as "hypoallergenic"), necklaces, medals, brooches, bracelets, watches, rings, anklets, and pins used for piercing ears or other parts of the body
Pure gold as weel, especially white gold, can contain nickel (yellow gold usually contains only a very low percentage). Silver is often used in a nickel alloy for costume jewelry, and patients are advised to refrain from wearing such jewelry
– **Industrial blending fluids**
Other objects in common use that contain nickel are:
– **Metal accessories for clothing:** bra hooks as well as eyes and other metal clasps in general, jeans buttons, zippers, belt and shoe buckles and studs, metal shoe inserts, safety pins, hairpins and hairclips, curling tongs, and eyelash curlers. Where possible, these objects should be replaced by their plastic, wood, or bone counterparts
– **Glasses with metal parts** (frames made of titanium are preferable)
– **Coins and keys** (these can cause "allergy" only after prolonged contact, e.g., in those working at the cash desks or if they are kept for long periods in a pocket). Metal keys, in particular, can be replaced by aluminum copies
– **Some cosmetics (especially mascara) and detergents used both for personal hygiene and at home** can contain traces of nickel
It is also important to avoid prolonged, repeated contact with some metal objects in domestic use that can contain nickel (pans, cutlery and other kitchen utensils, scissors, thimbles, needles, and pins), as well as contact with all metal handles, paper weights, razors, combs, curlers, pencil cases, lighters, as well as handbag and umbrella handles, musical instruments, and chairs with a metal frame

Alternative objects includes substitutes made of **stainless steel** and also **titanium, copper, and bronze**, which have a very low nickel content. It is always wise to wear **gloves** when doing housework, but avoid direct contact with rubber gloves by wearing vinyl gloves underneath, or **cotton** gloves when possible. **Stainless steel** does not generally cause problems, but it is better to use aluminum or Teflon pans, because some chemical-physical conditions occuring while food is cooking can foster the release of nickel from the steel alloy. Some foods, like canned products, can contain nickel; however, only in particular cases a special low-canned-food diet is recommended.

In cases requiring dental or orthopedic **prostheses**, a pacemaker, or cardiac valves, the doctor should be informed about any nickel allergy to insure the employment of nickel-free products.

Other Techniques of Diagnosis

Gianni Angelini and Eustachio Nettis

6.1 Semi-Open Test

The semi-open test is useful for testing products with suspected irritant properties supplied by the patient. A small amount (15 µl) of the product is applied with a cotton swab on an area (1 cm^2) of the skin and then covered with permeable tape (e.g., Scanpor®). Readings are performed in the same way as for patch testing.

6.2 Open Test

This is a non-occlusive test: the allergenic material, as is or dissolved in water or another solvent (ethanol, acetone, ether), is applied to the skin, usually on the inner face of the forearm. An open test is recommended as the first step when testing unknown or poorly defined products like those supplied by the patient. Such products are tested as is or dissolved in concentrations not exceeding 5%. Just 0.1–0.2 ml of the solution is applied, on a skin surface of 2 cm^2 or more. Readings are performed in the same way as for patch testing. A negative result to an open test is an indication to specialists that they can proceed with patch tests.

G. Angelini
Dermatology, University of Bari "Aldo Moro", Bari, Italy
e-mail: gianniang@alice.it

E. Nettis (✉)
Department of Emergency and Organ Transplantation, University of Bari "Aldo Moro", Bari, Italy
e-mail: ambulatorio.allergologia@uniba.it

© Springer Nature Switzerland AG 2020
E. Nettis, G. Angelini (eds.), *Practical Guide to Patch Testing*,
https://doi.org/10.1007/978-3-030-33873-2_6

6.3 Repeated Open Application Test (ROAT)

Commercially available products as is (cosmetics, topical drugs), or special substances used as a vehicle at suitable concentrations for patch tests, in quantities of 0.1 ml, are applied twice a day for 7 or more days on the inner surface of the forearm over an area of 1–5 cm^2 of healthy skin. If a positive erythematous-vesicular response appears, the test must be interrupted. The ROAT is used to clarify the relevance of some selected positive and doubtful patch test reactions.

Examples of Patch Test Reactions and Related 72-h Readings

Gianni Angelini and Eustachio Nettis

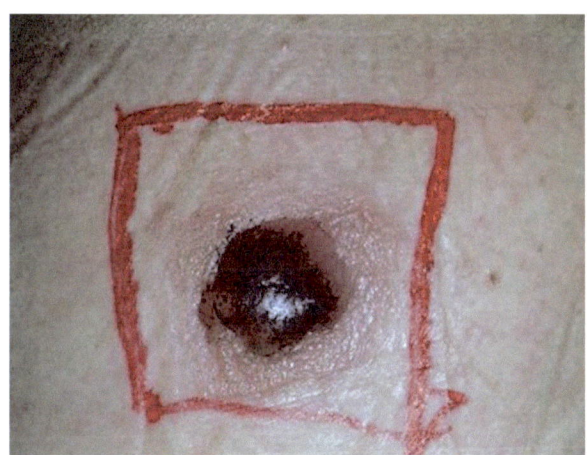

Fig. 7.1 Positive reaction, allergic: + + +. **Symptoms**: Pruritus. **Borders**: Irregular, blurred, extending beyond the hapten contact area. **Structure**: Homogeneous all over the test area. **Morphology**: Erythema, edema, evident papules, and vesicles confluent forming blisters. **Evolution**: "Increasing severity" reaction

---

G. Angelini
Dermatology, University of Bari "Aldo Moro", Bari, Italy
e-mail: gianniang@alice.it

E. Nettis (✉)
Department of Emergency and Organ Transplantation, University of Bari "Aldo Moro", Bari, Italy
e-mail: ambulatorio.allergologia@uniba.it

© Springer Nature Switzerland AG 2020
E. Nettis, G. Angelini (eds.), *Practical Guide to Patch Testing*,
https://doi.org/10.1007/978-3-030-33873-2_7

Fig. 7.2 Positive reaction, allergic: + + +. **Symptoms**: Pruritus. **Borders**: Irregular, blurred, extending beyond the hapten contact area. **Structure**: Homogeneous all over the test area. **Morphology**: Erythema, edema, evident papules, and vesicles. **Evolution**: "Increasing severity" reaction

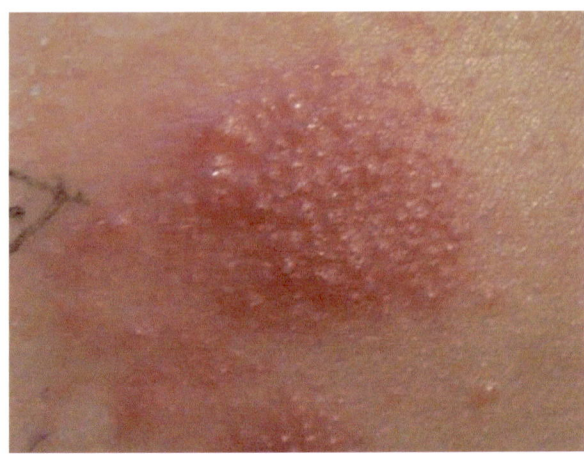

Fig. 7.3 Positive reaction, allergic: + +. **Symptoms**: Pruritus. **Borders**: Irregular, only slightly blurred, extending well beyond the hapten contact area. **Structure**: Homogeneous all over the test area. **Morphology**: Erythema, edema, a few evident papules, and vesicles. **Evolution**: "Increasing severity" reaction

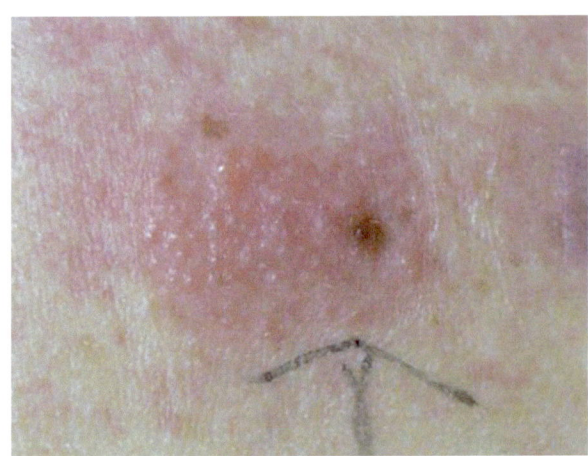

Fig. 7.4 Positive reaction, allergic: + +. **Symptoms**: Pruritus. **Borders**: Irregular, blurred, not extending beyond the hapten contact area. **Structure**: Nonhomogeneous over the test area. **Morphology**: Erythema, edema, some evident papules, and blisters. **Evolution**: "Increasing severity" reaction

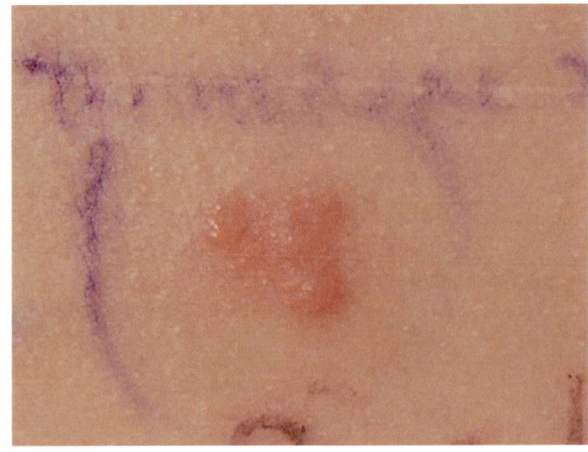

Fig. 7.5 Positive reaction, allergic: + + +. **Symptoms**: Pruritus. **Borders**: Irregular, blurred, extending well beyond the hapten contact area. **Structure**: Homogeneous all over the test area. **Morphology**: Erythema, edema, some papules, very evident vesicles, sometimes confluent forming blisters. **Evolution**: "Increasing severity" reaction

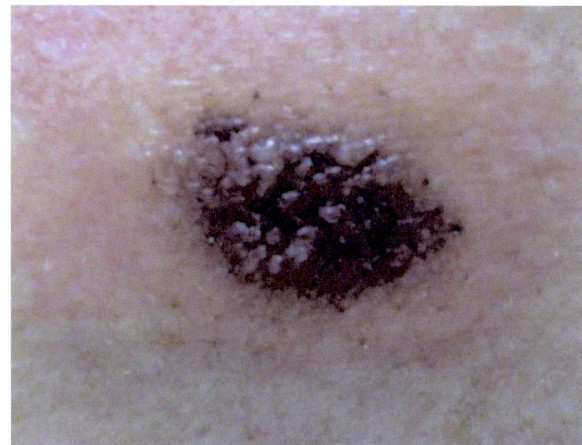

Fig. 7.6 Doubtful reaction. Nonhomogeneous erythema (the test should be repeated). **Symptoms**: None. **Borders**: Irregular, blurred, not extending beyond the hapten contact area. **Structure**: Nonhomogeneous over the test area. **Morphology**: Erythema

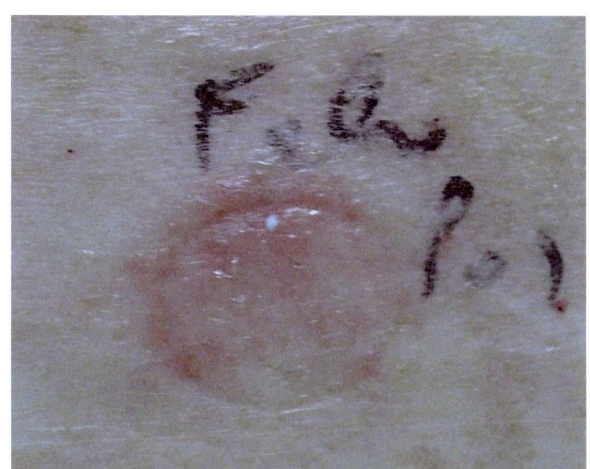

Fig. 7.7 Positive reaction, allergic: + + +. **Symptoms**: Pruritus. **Borders**: Irregular, blurred, and extending beyond the hapten contact area. **Structure**: Homogeneous all over the test area. **Morphology**: Erythema, edema, very evident vesicles, confluent forming blisters. **Evolution**: "Increasing severity" reaction

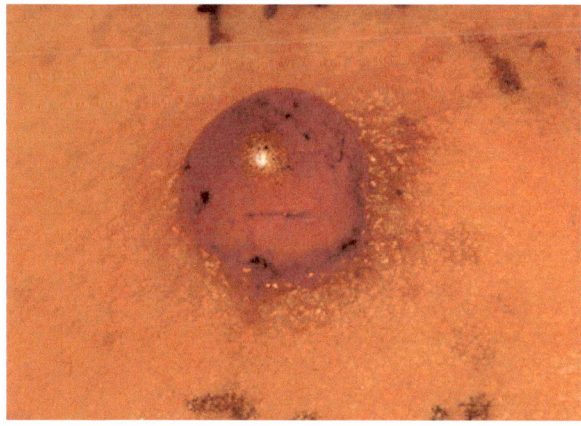

Fig. 7.8 Positive reaction, allergic: + + +. **Symptoms**: Pruritus. **Borders**: Irregular, blurred, extending well beyond the hapten contact area. **Structure**: Homogeneous all over the test area. **Morphology**: Erythema, edema, evident papules, and vesicles (prevalently vesicles). Evolution: "Increasing severity" reaction

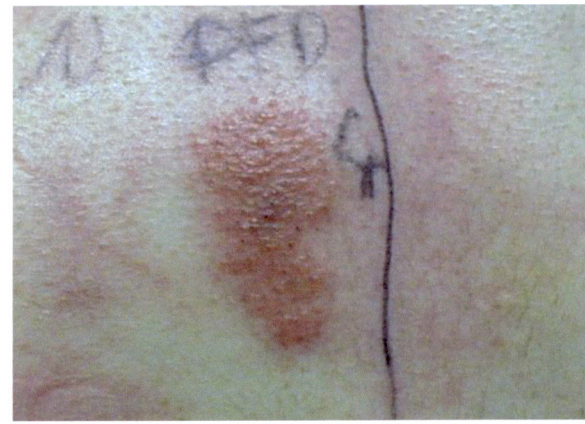

Fig. 7.9 Positive reaction, allergic: + +. **Symptoms**: Pruritus. **Borders**: Regular, fairly distinct, and not extending beyond the hapten contact area. **Structure**: Homogeneous all over the test area. **Morphology**: Erythema, edema, some papules, and a tendency to form vesicles. **Evolution**: "Increasing severity" reaction

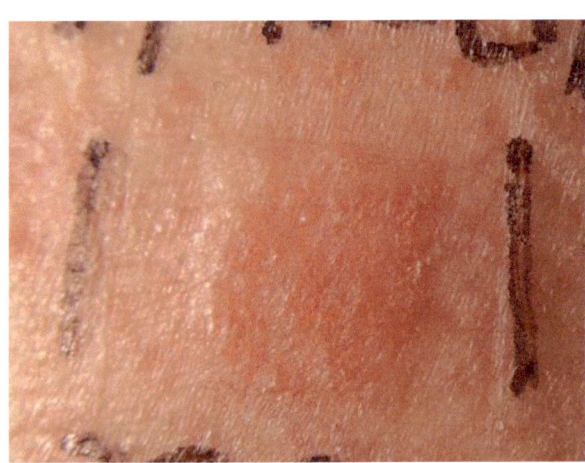

Fig. 7.10 Doubtful reaction. Nonhomogeneous erythema (the test should be repeated). **Symptoms**: None. **Borders**: Irregular, blurred not extending beyond the hapten contact area. **Structure**: Nonhomogeneous over the test area. **Morphology**: Erythema

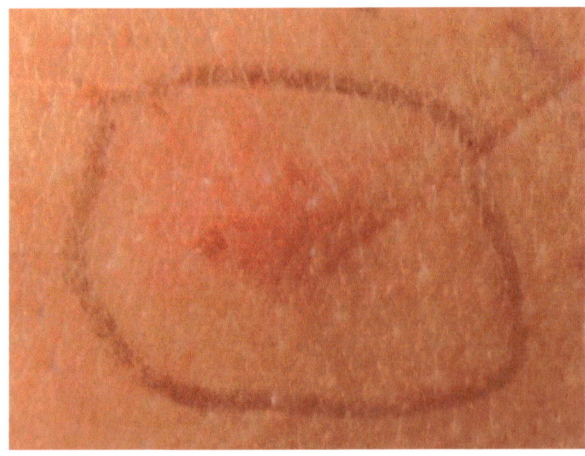

Fig. 7.11 Positive reaction, allergic: + +. **Symptoms**: Pruritus. **Borders**: Irregular, blurred, not extending beyond the hapten contact area. **Structure**: Homogeneous all over the test area. **Morphology**: Erythema, edema, evident papules, and vesicles (prevalently vesicles). **Evolution**: "Increasing severity" reaction

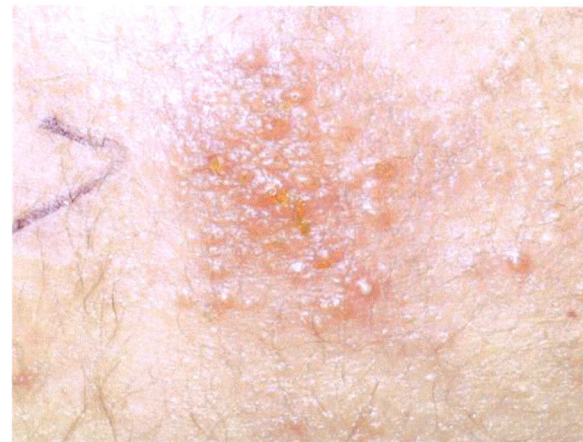

Fig. 7.12 False-positive reaction: papulous, follicular. Symptoms: None. **Borders**: Irregular, blurred. **Structure**: Nonhomogeneous over the test area. **Morphology**: Scattered brownish papules and vesicles. **Evolution**: "Decreasing severity" reaction

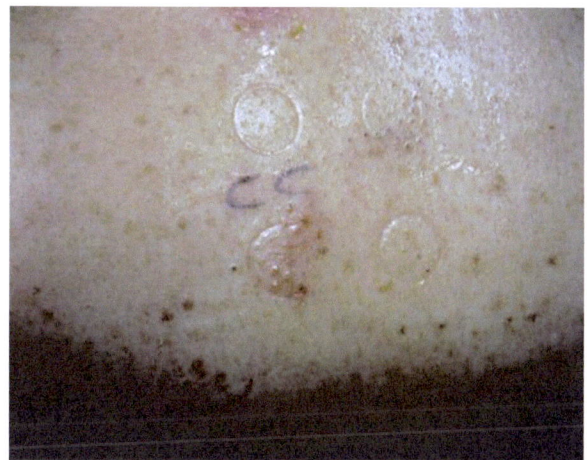

Fig. 7.13 Positive reaction, allergic: + +. **Symptoms**: Pruritus. **Borders**: Regular, distinct, not extending beyond the hapten contact area. **Structure**: Homogeneous all over the test area. **Morphology**: Erythema, edema, some papules, and evident vesicles. **Evolution**: "Increasing severity" reaction

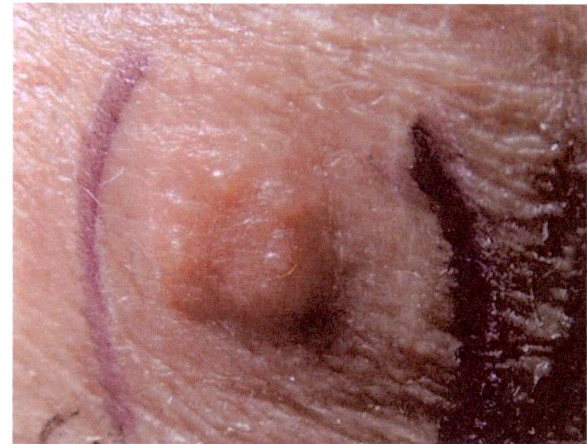

Fig. 7.14 Positive reaction, allergic: +. **Symptoms**: Pruritus. **Borders**: Regular, distinct, partly extending beyond the hapten contact area. **Structure**: Homogeneous all over the test area. **Morphology**: Erythema, edema, a few papules. **Evolution**: "Increasing severity" reaction

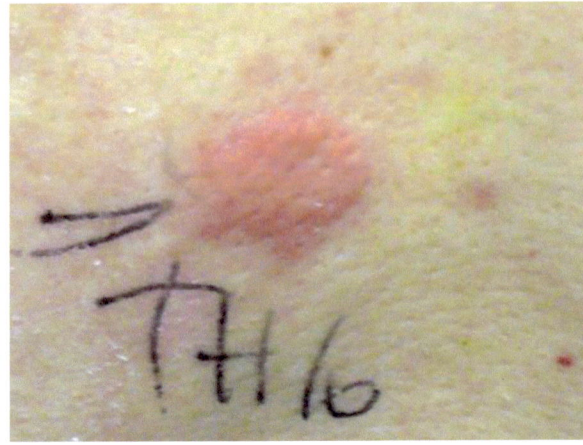

Fig. 7.15 False-positive reaction: "soap effect." **Symptoms**: A feeling of tension. **Borders**: Fairly irregular, fairly distinct. **Structure**: Homogeneous all over the test area. **Morphology**: Mild erythema with accentuated skin folds. **Evolution**: "Decreasing severity" reaction

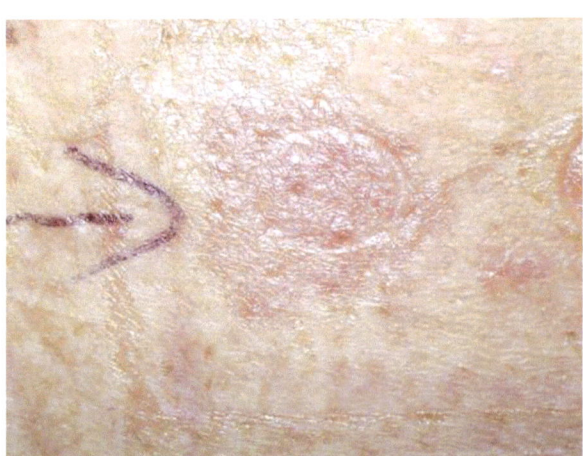

Fig. 7.16 Positive reaction, allergic: + +. **Symptoms**: Pruritus. **Borders**: Irregular, blurred, extending well beyond the hapten contact area. **Structure**: Homogeneous all over the test area. **Morphology**: Erythema, edema, evident papules, and vesicles (prevalently vesicles). **Evolution**: "Increasing severity" reaction

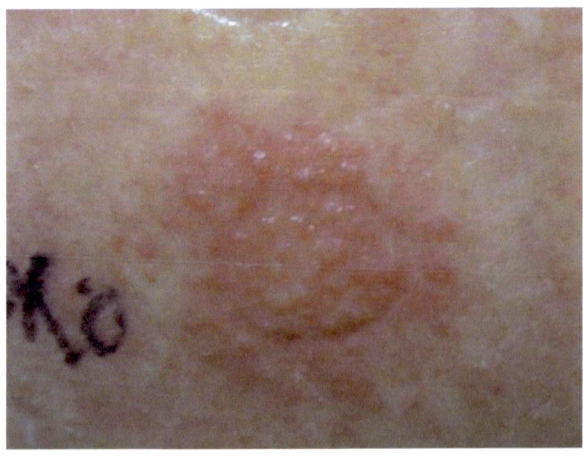

7 Examples of Patch Test Reactions and Related 72-h Readings 51

Fig. 7.17 Mixed reaction (the test should be repeated). **Symptoms**: Mild pruritus. **Borders**: Irregular, blurred, extending slightly beyond the hapten contact area. **Structure**: Homogeneous all over the test area. **Morphology**: Erythema, edema, papules, and vesicles as well as some pustules

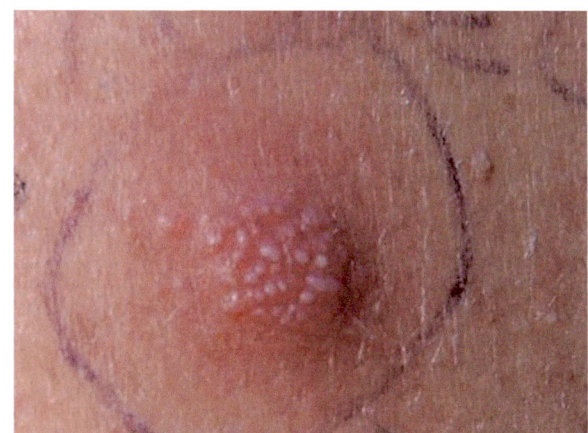

Fig. 7.18 Positive reaction, allergic: + + (reaction to nickel sulfate present in lip liners used in extemporaneous patch test). **Symptoms**: Pruritus. **Borders**: Fairly irregular and blurred, not extending beyond the hapten contact area. **Structure**: Homogeneous all over the test area. **Morphology**: Erythema, edema, some evident papules, and vesicles. **Evolution**: "Increasing severity" reaction

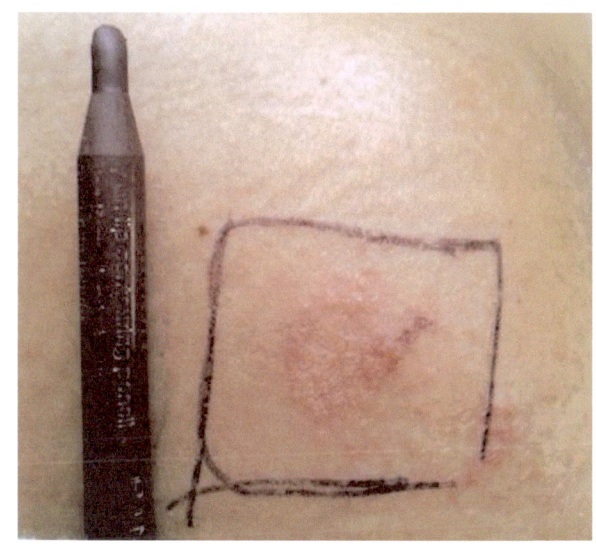

Fig. 7.19 Doubtful reaction: Homogeneous erythema (the test should be repeated). **Symptoms**: Mild pruritus. **Borders**: Regular, distinct, not extending beyond the hapten contact area. **Structure**: Homogeneous all over the test area. **Morphology**: Erythema

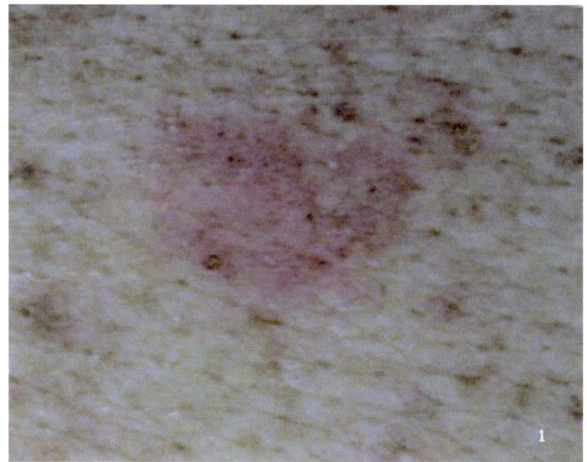

Fig. 7.20 Positive reaction, allergic: + + (reaction to dust mites present in additional atopy series—inhalants). **Symptoms**: Pruritus. **Borders**: Slightly irregular, fairly distinct, extending well beyond the hapten contact area. **Structure**: Homogeneous all over the test area. **Morphology**: Erythema, edema, some evident papules, and vesicles (prevalently vesicles). **Evolution**: "Increasing severity" reaction

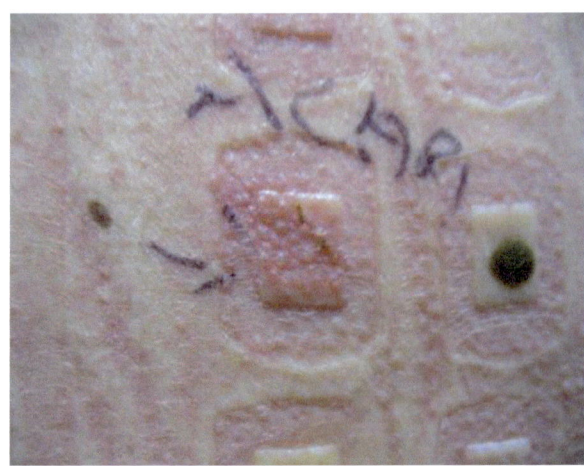

Fig. 7.21 False-positive reaction: pustulous. **Symptoms**: None. **Borders**: Irregular, blurred. **Structure**: Nonhomogeneous over the test area. **Morphology**: A few papules, numerous pustules with a slightly erythematous base. **Evolution**: "Decreasing severity" reaction

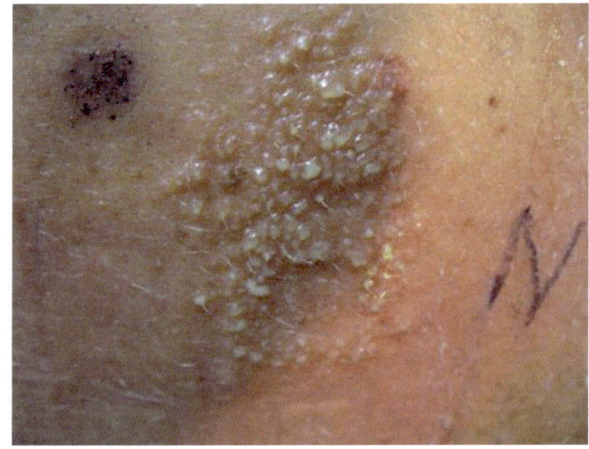

Fig. 7.22 Positive reaction, allergic: +. **Symptoms**: Pruritus. **Borders**: Slightly irregular, blurred but not extending beyond the hapten contact area. **Structure**: Homogeneous all over the test area. **Morphology**: Erythema, edema, a few papules, and a tendency to form vesicles. **Evolution**: "Increasing severity" reaction

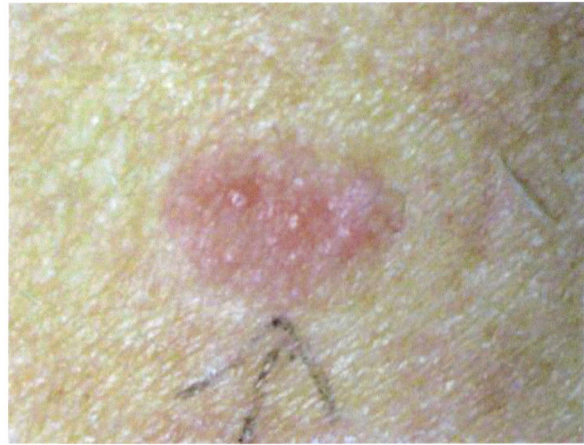

7 Examples of Patch Test Reactions and Related 72-h Readings

Fig. 7.23 Positive reaction, allergic: + + +. **Symptoms**: Pruritus. **Borders**: Regular, quite distinct, and not extending beyond the hapten contact area. **Structure**: Homogeneous all over the test area. **Morphology**: Erythema, edema, a few papules, very evident vesicles, sometimes confluent forming blisters. **Evolution**: "Increasing severity" reaction

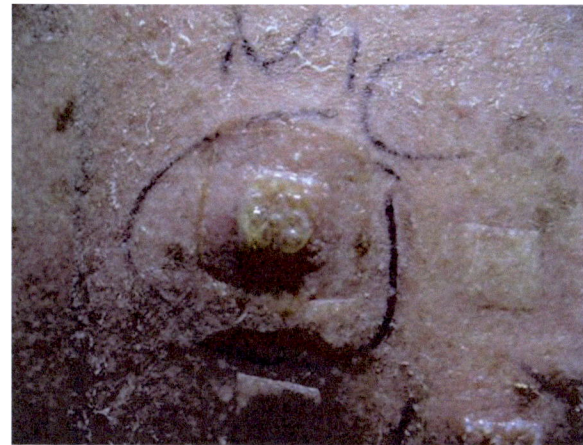

Fig. 7.24 False-positive reaction: papulous, follicular. **Symptoms**: Pruritus. **Borders**: Regular, quite distinct, and not extending beyond the hapten contact area. **Structure**: Homogeneous all over the test area. **Morphology**: Erythema, edema, a few papules, very evident vesicles, sometimes confluent forming blisters. **Evolution**: "Increasing severity" reaction

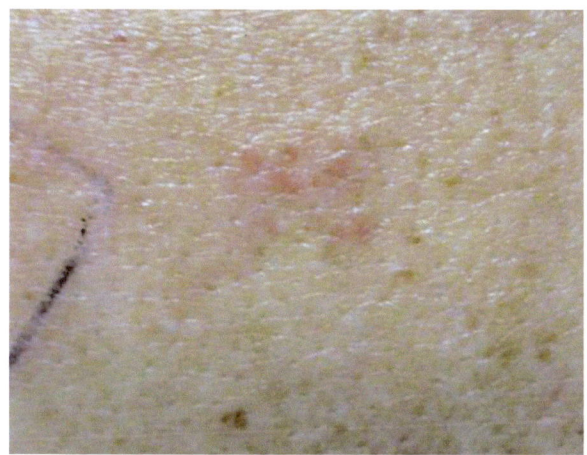

Fig. 7.25 Positive reaction, allergic: + + +. **Symptoms**: Pruritus. **Borders**: Fairly irregular, minor blurring, and extending only slightly beyond the hapten contact area. **Structure**: Homogeneous all over the test area. **Morphology**: Erythema, edema, very evident papules, and vesicles, sometimes confluent forming blisters. **Evolution**: "Increasing severity" reaction

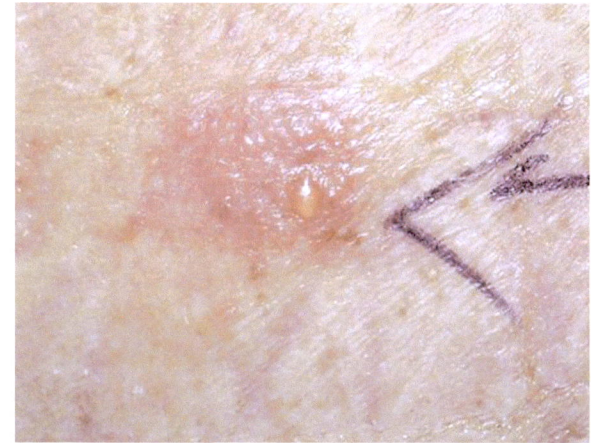

Fig. 7.26 False-positive reaction: "border" effect. Erythematous ring, purpuric at the periphery of the test area. **Evolution**: "Decreasing severity" reaction

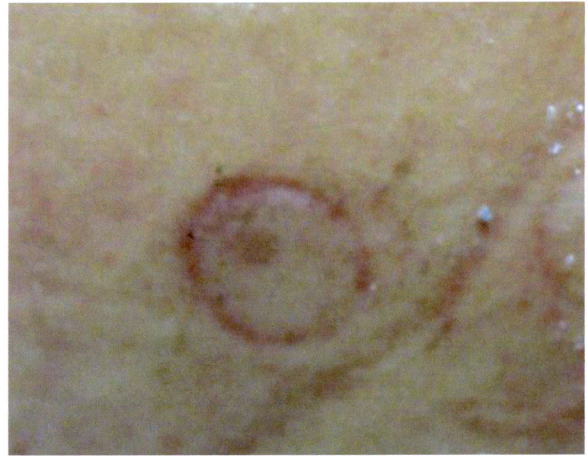

Fig. 7.27 "Excited skin syndrome"

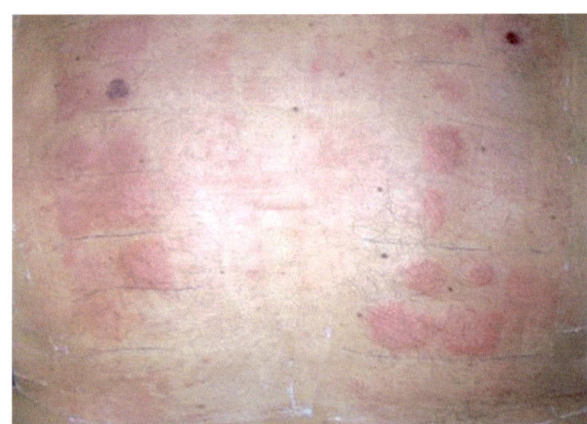

Fig. 7.28 Positive reaction, allergic: + +. **Symptoms**: Pruritus. **Borders**: Irregular, blurred, extending well beyond the hapten contact area. **Structure**: Homogeneous all over the test area. **Morphology**: Erythema, edema, evident papules, and vesicles (prevalently vesicles). **Evolution**: "Increasing severity" reaction

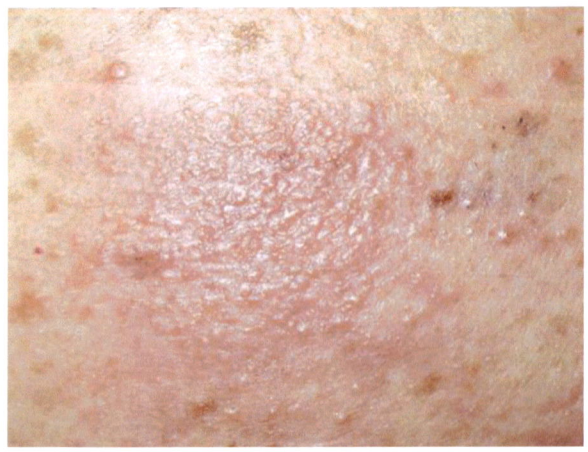

7 Examples of Patch Test Reactions and Related 72-h Readings

Fig. 7.29 Positive reaction, allergic: + + +. **Symptoms**: Pruritus. **Borders**: Irregular, blurred, extending well beyond the hapten contact area. **Structure**: Homogeneous all over the test area. **Morphology**: Erythema, edema, evident papules, and vesicles (prevalently vesicles). **Evolution**: "Increasing severity" reaction

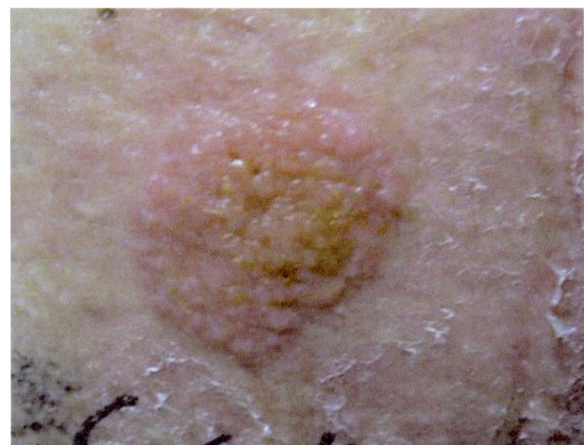

Fig. 7.30 False-positive reaction: bullous. **Symptoms**: None. **Borders**: Distinct and not extending beyond the hapten contact area. **Structure**: Homogeneous all over the test area. **Morphology**: Blisters, not preceded by vesicles. **Evolution**: "Increasing severity" reaction

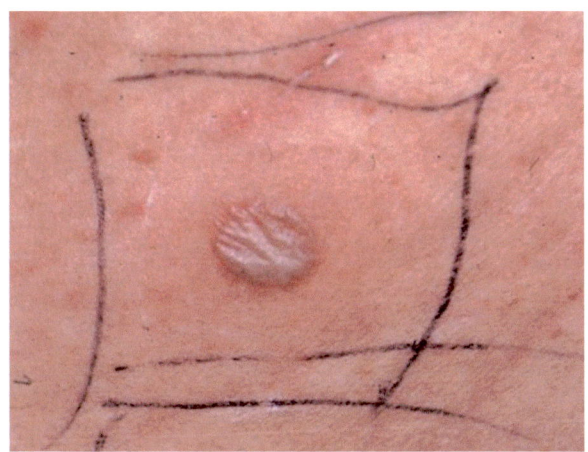

Fig. 7.31 Positive reaction, allergic: + +. **Symptoms**: Pruritus. **Borders**: Irregular, blurred, extending well beyond the hapten contact area. **Structure**: Homogeneous all over the test area. **Morphology**: Erythema, edema, evident papules, and vesicles (prevalently vesicles). **Evolution**: "Increasing severity" reaction

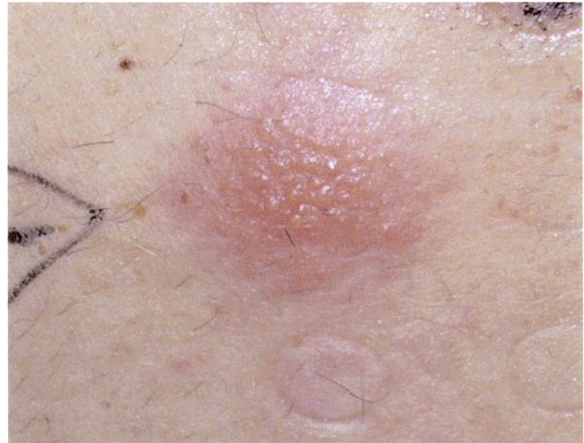

Fig. 7.32 False-positive reaction: Erythemato-purpuric. **Symptoms**: None. **Borders**: Poorly defined. **Structure**: Nonhomogeneous over the test area. **Morphology**: Mild erythema and small reddish-purple papules. **Evolution**: "Decreasing severity" reaction

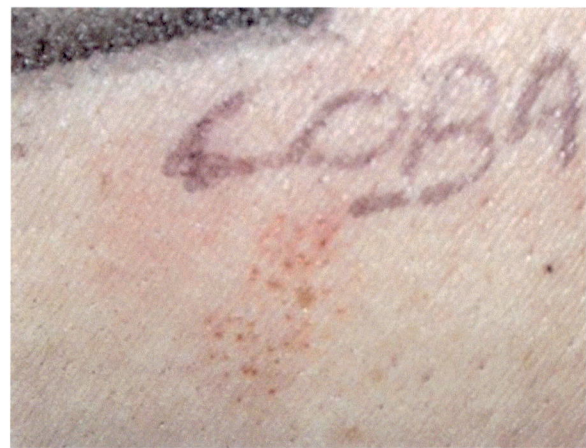

Fig. 7.33 Positive reaction, allergic: + + +. **Symptoms**: Pruritus. **Borders**: Irregular, blurred, extending well beyond the hapten contact area. **Structure**: Homogeneous all over the test area. **Morphology**: Erythema, edema, a few papules, very evident vesicles, sometimes confluent forming blisters. **Evolution**: "Increasing severity" reaction

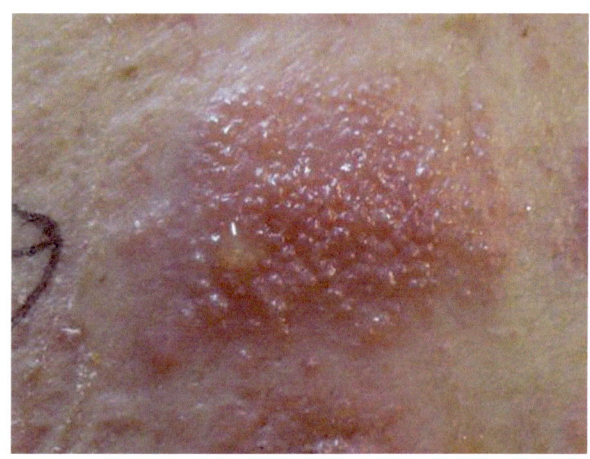

Fig. 7.34 Positive reaction, allergic: +. **Symptoms**: Pruritus. **Borders**: Slightly irregular, faintly blurred, and extending beyond the hapten contact area. **Structure**: Homogeneous all over the test area. **Morphology**: Erythema, edema, a few papules, and a tendency to form vesicles. **Evolution**: "Increasing severity" reaction

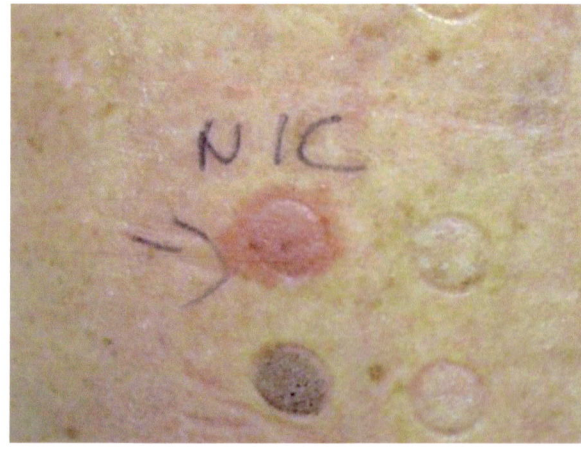

7 Examples of Patch Test Reactions and Related 72-h Readings

Fig. 7.35 Mixed reaction (the test should be repeated). **Symptoms**: Mild pruritus. **Borders**: Irregular, blurred, extending beyond the hapten contact area. **Structure**: Nonhomogeneous over the test area. **Morphology**: Erythema, edema, papules, a few vesicles, and some pustules

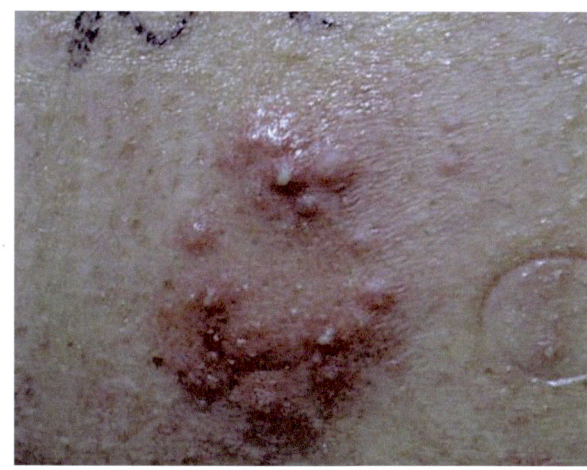

Fig. 7.36 Positive reaction, allergic: + +. **Symptoms**: Pruritus. **Borders**: Irregular, blurred, extending well beyond the hapten contact area. **Structure**: Homogeneous all over the test area. **Morphology**: Erythema, edema, evident papules, and vesicles (prevalently vesicles). **Evolution**: "Increasing severity" reaction

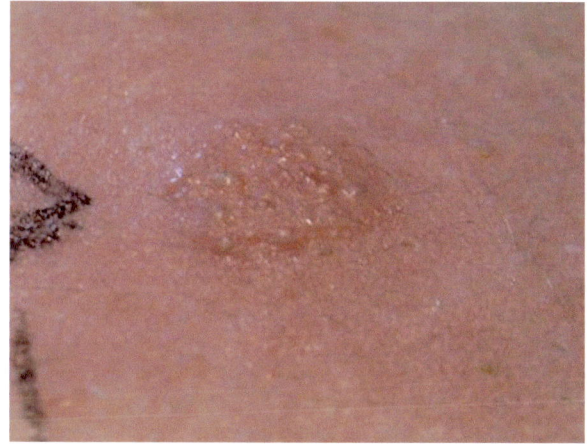

Fig. 7.37 False-positive reaction: papulous, follicular. **Symptoms**: None. **Borders**: Slightly irregular, distinct, and confined to the test area. **Structure**: Nonhomogeneous over the test area. **Morphology**: Mild erythema and some papules. **Evolution**: "Decreasing severity" reaction

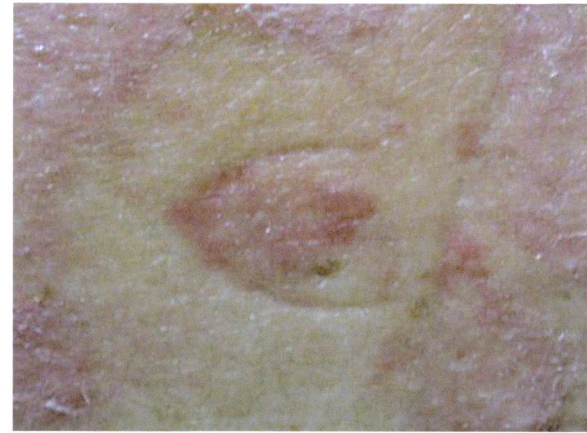

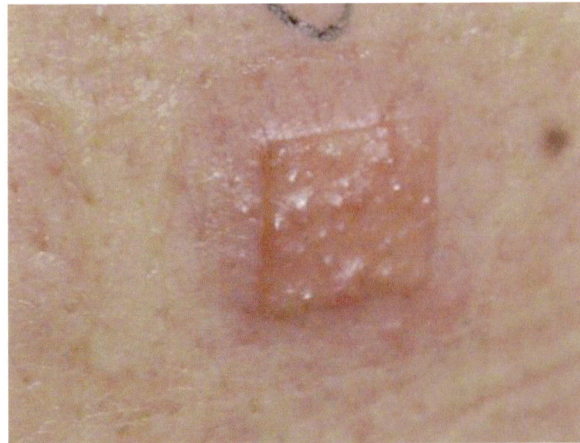

Fig. 7.38 Positive reaction, allergic: + +. **Symptoms**: Pruritus. **Borders**: Irregular, blurred, extending well beyond the hapten contact area. **Structure**: Homogeneous all over the test area. **Morphology**: Erythema, edema, some evident papules, and vesicles. **Evolution**: "Increasing severity" reaction

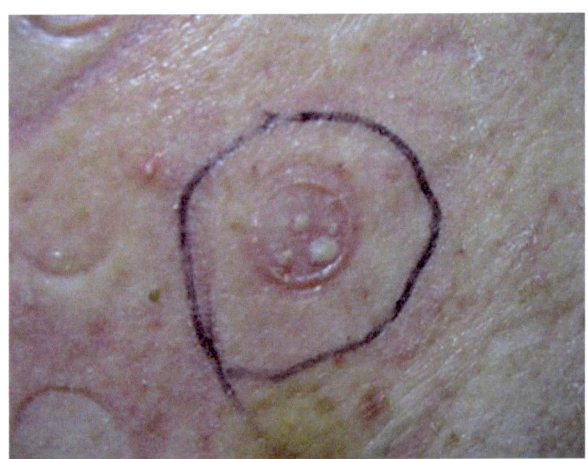

Fig. 7.39 False-positive reaction. **Symptoms**: None. **Borders**: Regular, distinct. **Structure**: Nonhomogeneous all over the test area. **Morphology**: Erythema, pustules with a "border effect." **Evolution**: "Decreasing severity" reaction

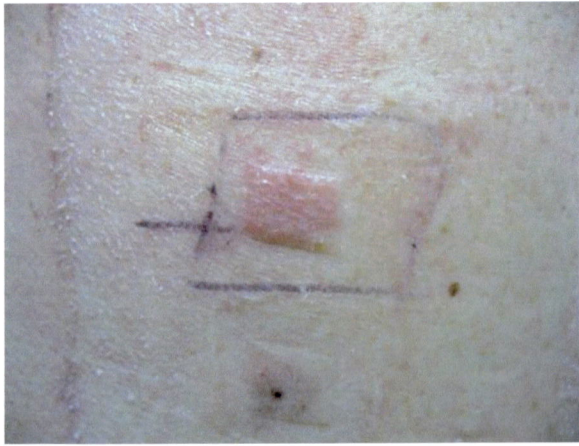

Fig. 7.40 Positive reaction, allergic to Kathon CG: +. **Symptoms**: Pruritus. **Borders**: Regular, distinct, not extending beyond the hapten contact area. **Structure**: Homogeneous all over the test area. **Morphology**: Mild erythema, edema, a few papules, and a tendency to form vesicles (the reaction to Kathon CG shows distinct margins and is confined to the application area). **Evolution**: "Increasing severity" reaction

7 Examples of Patch Test Reactions and Related 72-h Readings 59

Fig. 7.41 Positive reaction, allergic: + + +. **Symptoms**: Pruritus. **Borders**: Slightly irregular, faintly blurred, and extending well beyond the hapten contact area. **Structure**: Homogeneous all over the test area. **Morphology**: Erythema, edema, a few papules, very evident vesicles, sometimes confluent forming blisters. **Evolution**: "Increasing severity" reaction

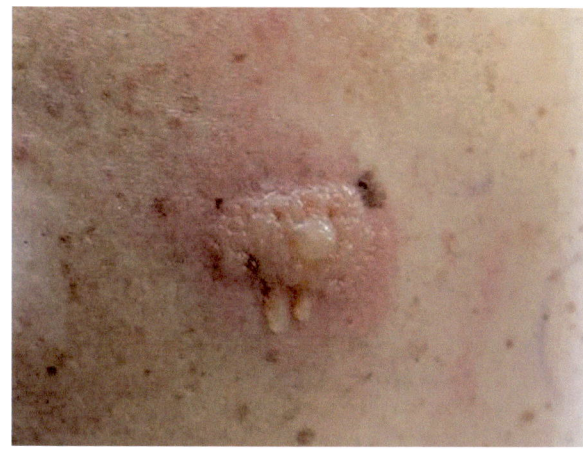

Fig. 7.42 Positive reaction, allergic: + + +. **Symptoms**: Pruritus. **Borders**: Irregular, blurred, extending well beyond the hapten contact area. **Structure**: Homogeneous all over the test area. **Morphology**: Erythema, edema, evident papules, and vesicles (prevalently vesicles). **Evolution**: "Increasing severity" reaction

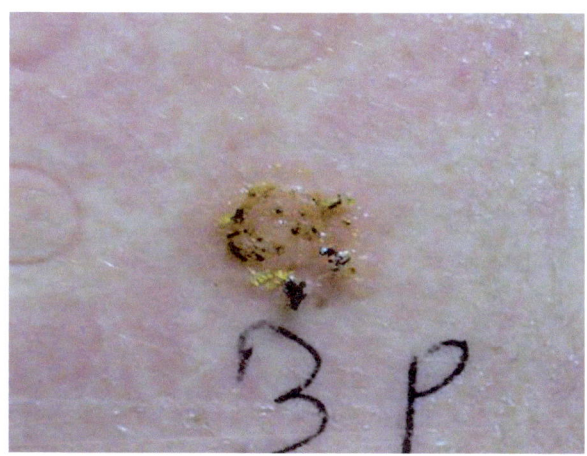

Fig. 7.43 Positive reaction, allergic: + + +. **Symptoms**: Pruritus. **Borders**: Irregular, slightly blurred, extending well beyond the hapten contact area. **Structure**: Homogeneous all over the test area. **Morphology**: Erythema, edema, a few papules, very evident vesicles, often confluent, forming blisters. **Evolution**: "Increasing severity" reaction

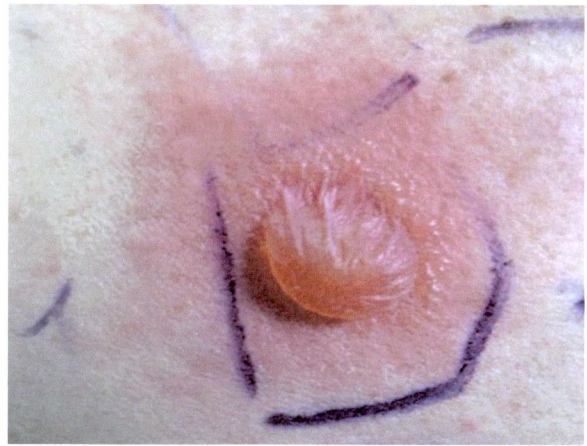

Fig. 7.44 False-positive reaction: papulous, follicular. Symptoms: None. **Borders**: Irregular, slightly blurred, not extending beyond the hapten contact area. **Structure**: Nonhomogeneous over the test area. **Morphology**: Mild erythema and follicular papules. **Evolution**: "Decreasing severity" reaction

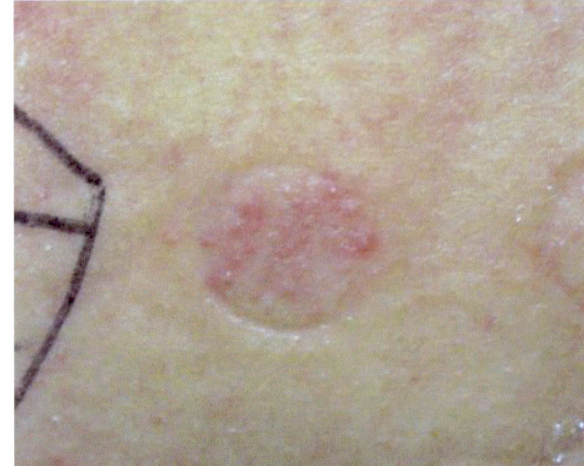

Fig. 7.45 Positive reaction, allergic to Kathon CG: + +. **Symptoms**: Pruritus. **Borders**: Regular, distinct, not extending beyond the hapten contact area. **Structure**: Homogeneous all over the test area. **Morphology**: Mild erythema, edema, some evident papules, and vesicles (the reaction to Kathon CG shows distinct margins and is confined to the application area). **Evolution**: "Increasing severity" reaction

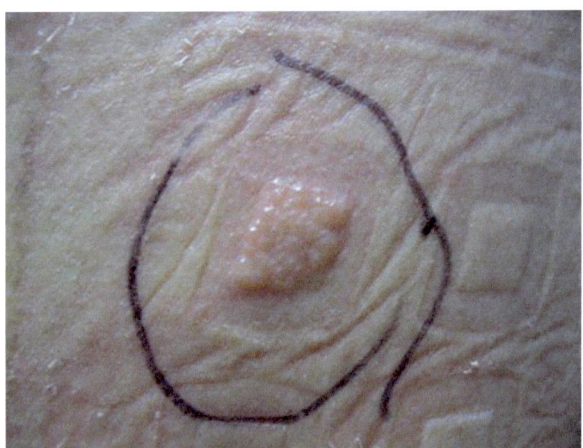

Fig. 7.46 Mixed reaction (the test should be repeated). **Symptoms**: Pruritus. **Borders**: Irregular, blurred, extending beyond the hapten contact area. **Structure**: Nonhomogeneous over the test area. **Morphology**: Erythema, a few papules, some vesicles, and pustules

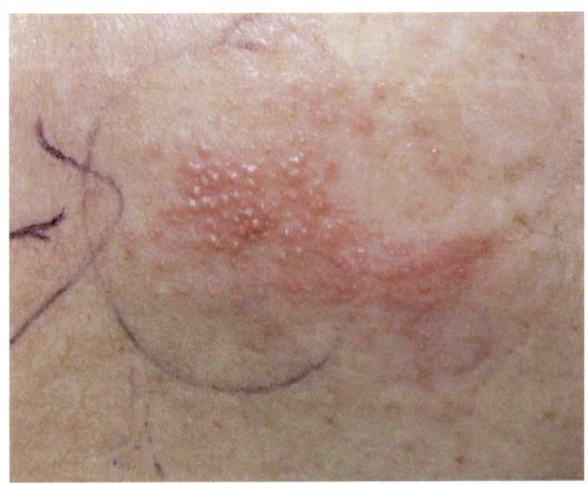

7 Examples of Patch Test Reactions and Related 72-h Readings

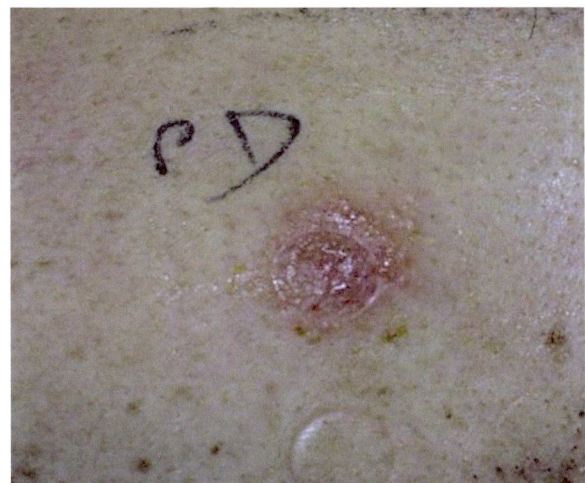

Fig. 7.47 Positive reaction, allergic: + +. **Symptoms**: Pruritus. **Borders**: Irregular, blurred, extending well beyond the hapten contact area. **Structure**: Homogeneous all over the test area. **Morphology**: Erythema, edema, evident papules, and vesicles (prevalently vesicles). **Evolution**: "Increasing severity" reaction

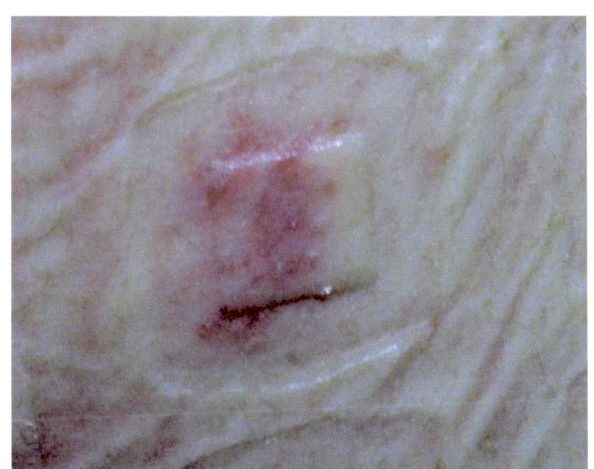

Fig. 7.48 False-positive reaction: papulous, follicular. **Symptoms**: None. **Borders**: Slightly irregular, faintly blurred, and partly extending beyond the hapten contact area. **Structure**: Nonhomogeneous over the test area. **Morphology**: Mild erythema and follicular papules. **Evolution**: "Decreasing severity" reaction

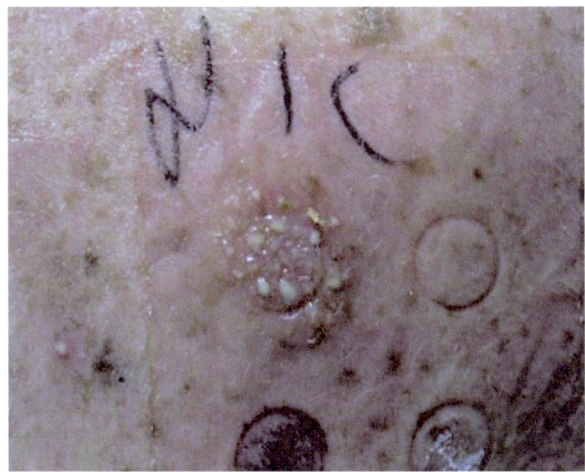

Fig. 7.49 False-positive reaction: pustulous. **Symptoms**: None. **Borders**: Irregular, blurred, extending beyond the hapten contact area. **Structure**: Nonhomogeneous over the test area. **Morphology**: A few papules, many pustules with a mildly erythematous base. **Evolution**: "Decreasing severity" reaction

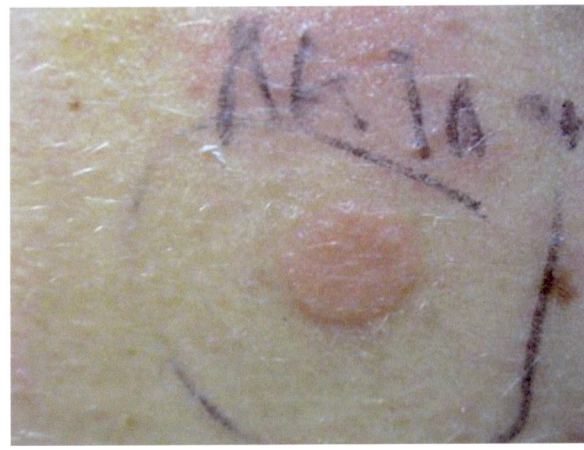

Fig. 7.50 Positive reaction, allergic to Kathon CG: +. **Symptoms**: Pruritus. **Borders**: Regular, distinct, not extending beyond the hapten contact area. **Structure**: Homogeneous all over the test area. **Morphology**: Mild erythema, edema, some evident papules, and vesicles (the reaction to Kathon CG shows distinct margins and is confined to the application area). **Evolution**: "Increasing severity" reaction

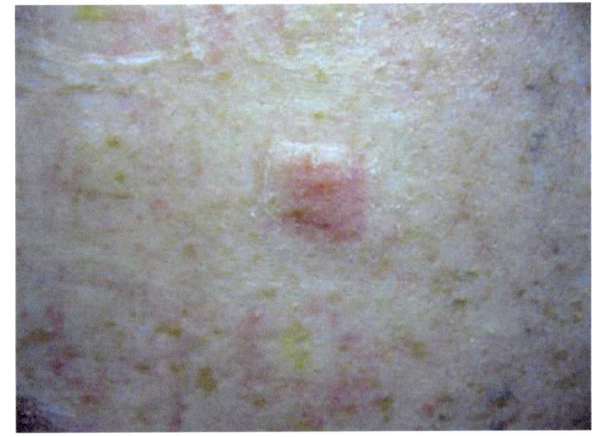

Fig. 7.51 Doubtful reaction: Homogeneous erythema (the test should be repeated). **Symptoms**: Mild pruritus. **Borders**: Regular, distinct, partly extending beyond the hapten contact area. **Structure**: Homogeneous all over the test area. **Morphology**: Erythema

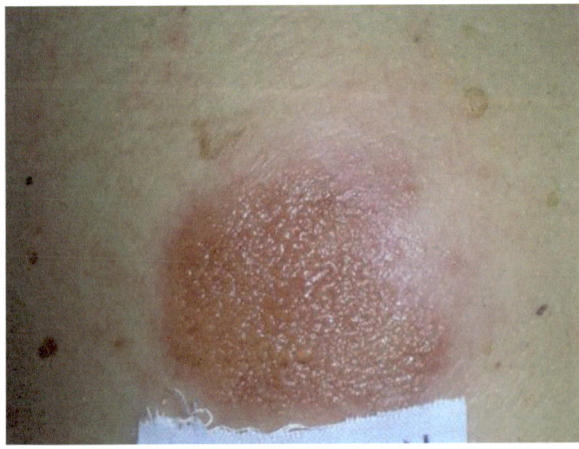

Fig. 7.52 Positive reaction, allergic: + + +. **Symptoms**: Pruritus. **Borders**: Slightly irregular, faintly blurred, extending well beyond the hapten contact area. **Structure**: Homogeneous all over the test area. **Morphology**: Erythema, edema, a few papules, very evident vesicles, sometimes confluent forming blisters. **Evolution**: "Increasing severity" reaction

Fig. 7.53 "Excited skin syndrome"

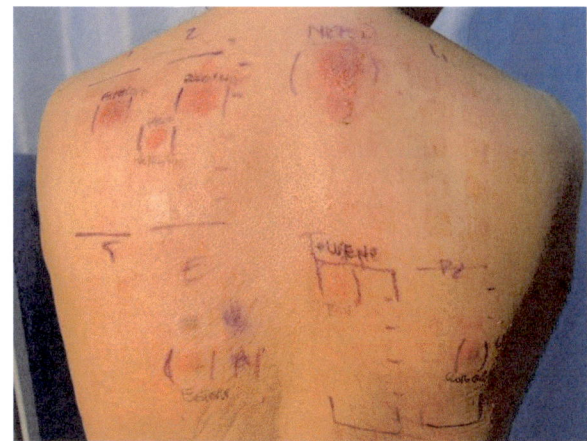

Fig. 7.54 Positive reaction, allergic: + + +. **Symptoms**: Pruritus. **Borders**: Irregular, slightly blurred, extending well beyond the hapten contact area. **Structure**: Homogeneous all over the test area. **Morphology**: Erythema, edema, a few papules, very evident vesicles, sometimes confluent forming blisters. **Evolution**: "Increasing severity" reaction

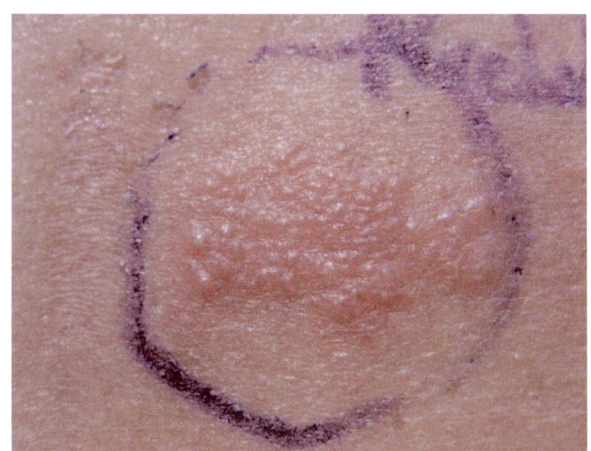

Fig. 7.55 Positive reaction, allergic to Kathon CG: + +. **Symptoms**: Pruritus. **Borders**: Regular, distinct, not extending beyond the hapten contact area. **Structure**: Homogeneous all over the test area. **Morphology**: Mild erythema, edema, some evident papules and vesicles (the reaction to Kathon CG shows distinct margins and is confined to the application area). **Evolution**: "Increasing severity" reaction

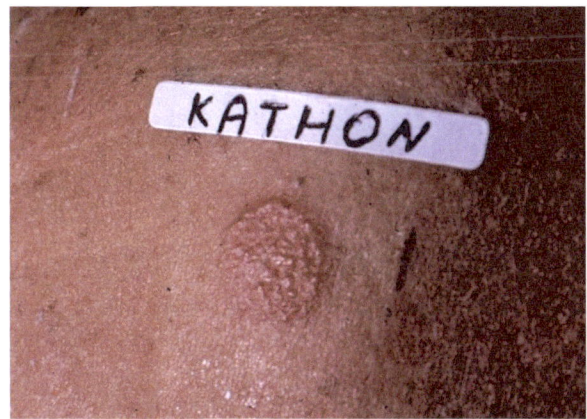

Fig. 7.56 Positive reaction, allergic: +. **Symptoms**: Pruritus. **Borders**: Irregular, faintly blurred, partly extending beyond the hapten contact area. **Structure**: Homogeneous all over the test area. **Morphology**: Erythema, edema, a few papules, and a tendency to form vesicles. **Evolution**: "Increasing severity" reaction

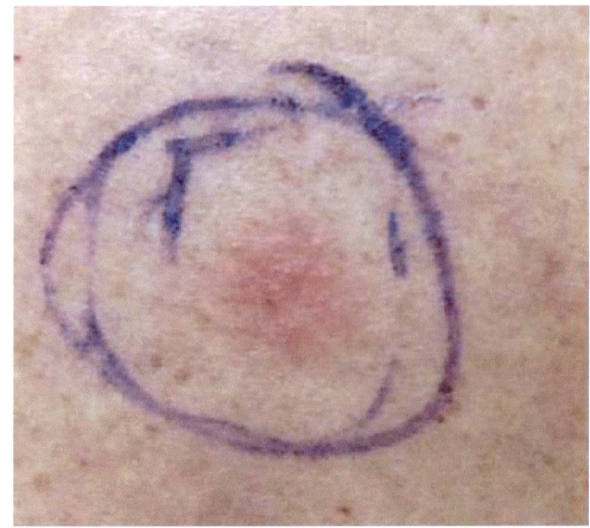

Fig. 7.57 Doubtful reaction: Nonhomogeneous erythema (the test should be repeated). **Symptoms**: None. **Borders**: Irregular, blurred, not extending beyond the hapten contact area. **Structure**: Nonhomogeneous over the test area. **Morphology**: Erytthema

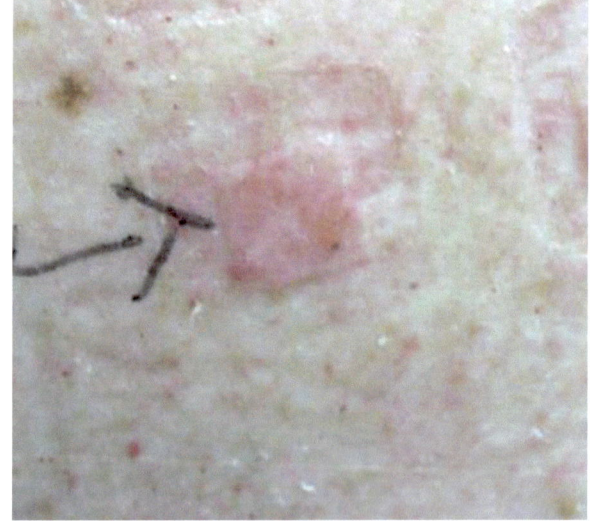

Fig. 7.58 False-positive reaction: pustulous. **Symptoms**: None. **Borders**: Slightly irregular, faintly blurred, not extending beyond the hapten contact area. **Structure**: Nonhomogeneous over the test area. **Morphology**: A few pustules with a mildly erythematous base. **Evolution**: "Decreasing severity" reaction

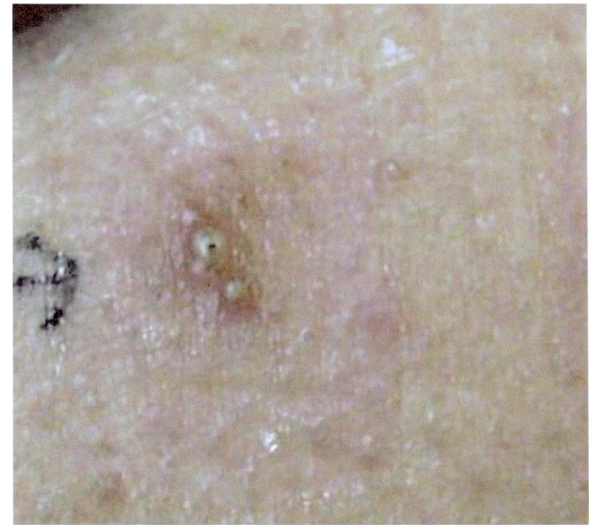

Fig. 7.59 False-positive reaction: pustulous. **Symptoms**: None. **Borders**: Irregular, blurred, partly extending beyond the hapten contact area. **Structure**: Nonhomogeneous over the test area. **Morphology**: A few pustules with an erythematous base. **Evolution**: "Decreasing severity" reaction

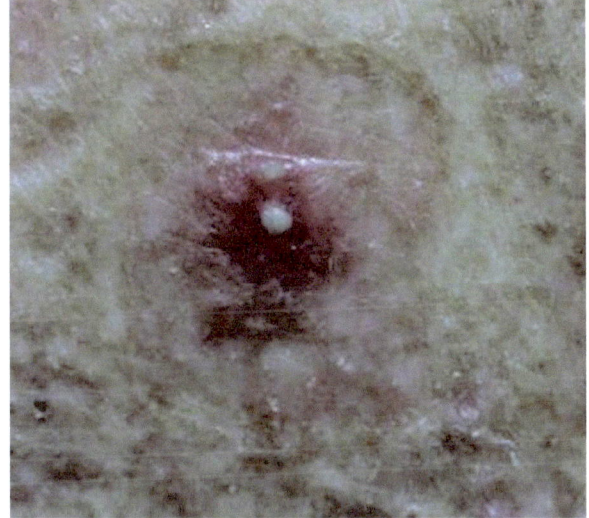

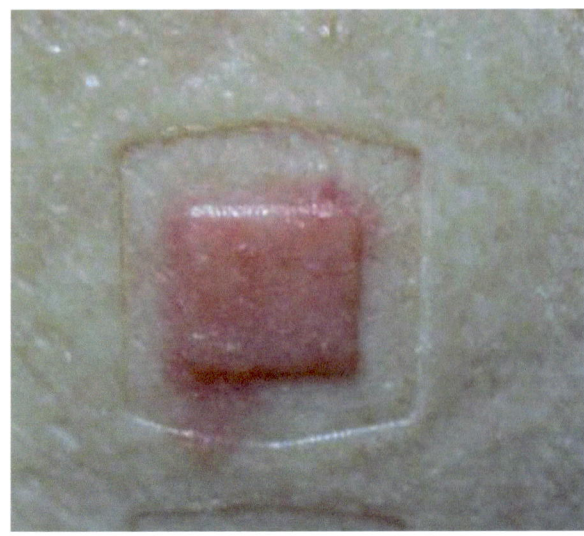

Fig. 7.60 Positive reaction, allergic to Kathon CG: +. **Symptoms**: Pruritus. **Borders**: Regular, distinct, not extending beyond the hapten contact area. **Structure**: Homogeneous all over the test area. **Morphology**: Mild erythema, edema, slight blistering (the reaction to Kathon CG shows distinct margins and is confined to the application area). **Evolution**: "Increasing severity" reaction

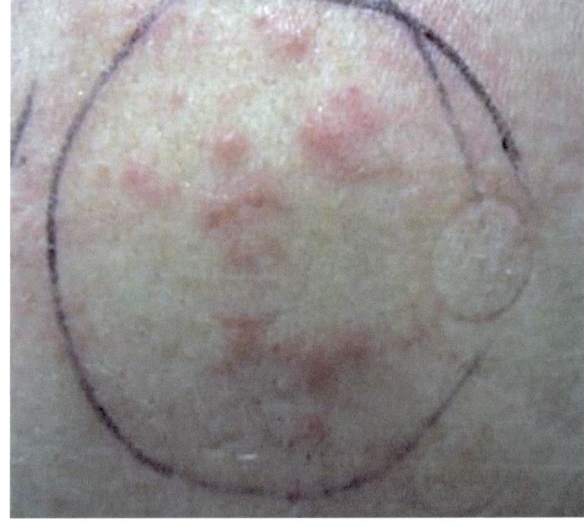

Fig. 7.61 False-positive reaction: papulous, follicular. **Symptoms**: None. **Borders**: Slightly irregular, faintly blurred. **Structure**: Nonhomogeneous all over the test area. **Morphology**: Mild erythema and follicular papules. **Evolution**: "Decreasing severity" reaction

Fig. 7.62 Positive reaction, allergic: + +. **Symptoms**: Pruritus. **Borders**: Irregular, slightly blurred, extending well beyond the hapten contact area. **Structure**: Homogeneous all over the test area. **Morphology**: Erythema, edema, a few papules, and evident vesicles. **Evolution**: "Increasing severity" reaction

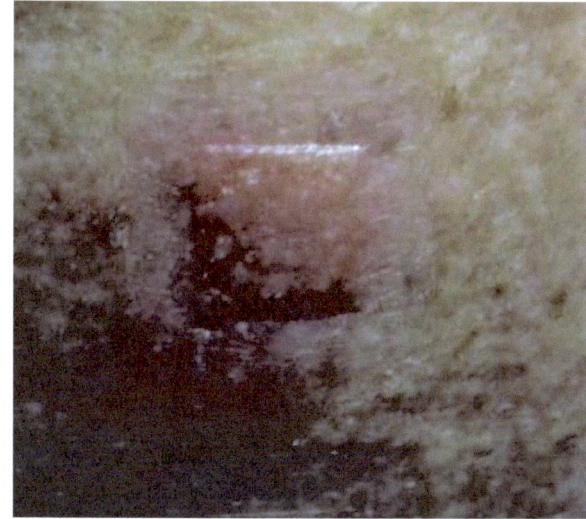

Fig. 7.63 Mixed reaction (the test should be repeated). **Symptoms**: Pruritus. **Borders**: Regular, faintly blurred, and extending slightly beyond the hapten contact area. **Structure**: Homogeneous all over the test area. **Morphology**: Erythema, edema, a few papules, some vesicles, and pustules

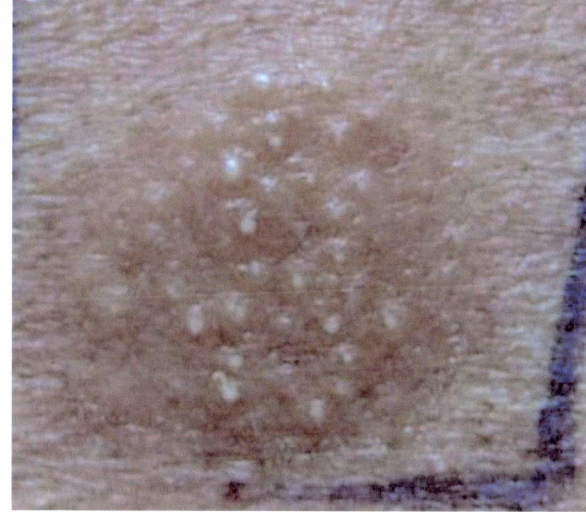

Fig. 7.64 Positive reaction, allergic: +. **Symptoms**: Pruritus. **Borders**: Irregular, blurred, extending beyond the hapten contact area. **Structure**: Homogeneous all over the test area. **Morphology**: Erythema, edema, a few papules, and a tendency to form vesicles. **Evolution**: "Increasing severity" reaction

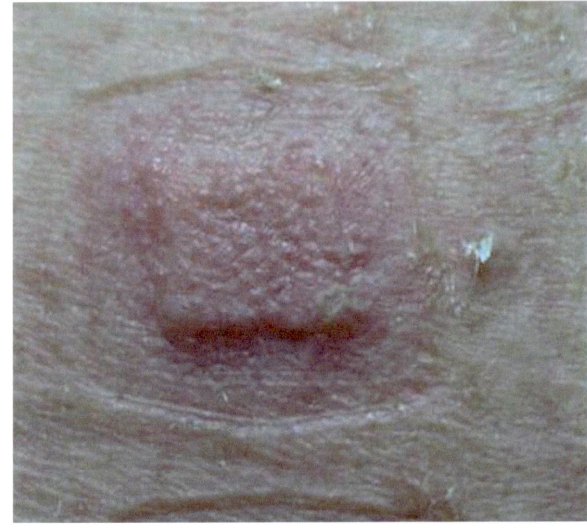

Fig. 7.65 Positive reaction, allergic: + +. **Symptoms**: Pruritus. **Borders**: Slightly irregular, blurred, and extending well byond the hapten contact area. **Structure**: Homogeneous all over the test area. **Morphology**: Erythema, edema, a few evident papules, and pustules. **Evolution**: "Increasing severity" reaction

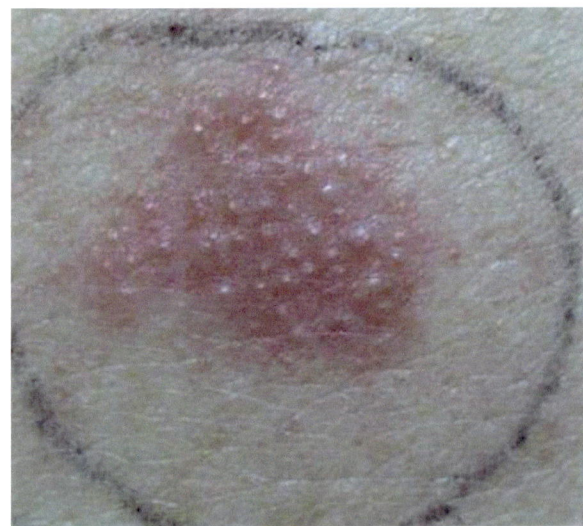

Fig. 7.66 Positive reaction, allergic: + + +. **Symptoms**: Pruritus. **Borders**: Irregular, slightly blurred, and extending well beyond the hapten contact area. **Structure**: Homogeneous all over the test area. **Morphology**: Erythema, edema, very evident papules, and vesicles, sometimes confluent forming blisters. **Evolution**: "Increasing severity" reaction

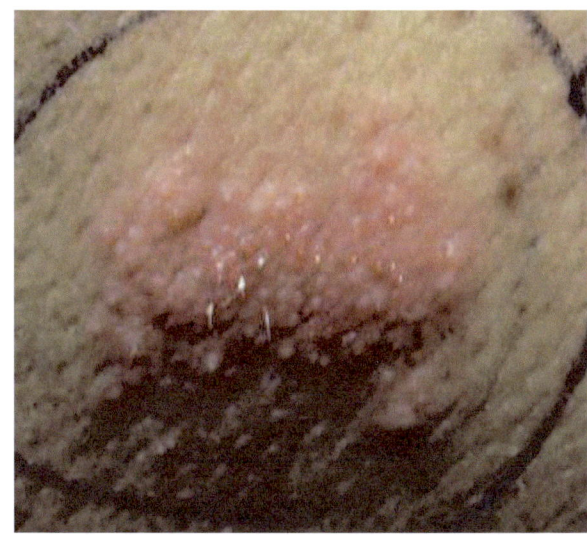

Fig. 7.67 Positive reaction, allergic: + + +. **Symptoms**: Pruritus. **Borders**: Slightly irregular, blurred, extending well beyond the hapten contact area. **Structure**: Homogeneous all over the test area. **Morphology**: Erythema, edema, very evident papules, and vesicles, sometimes confluent forming blisters. **Evolution**: "Increasing severity" reaction

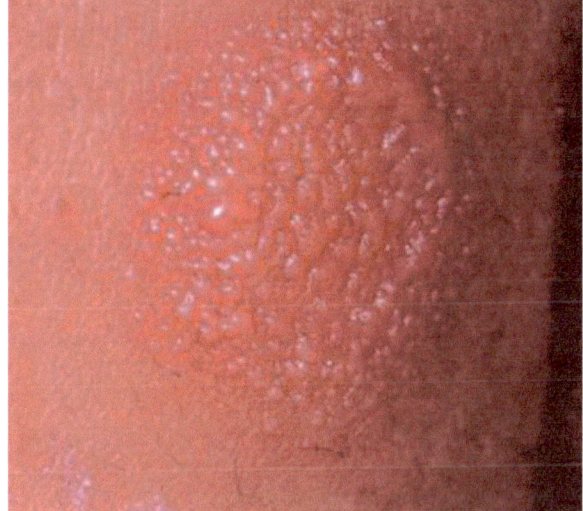

Fig. 7.68 Positive reaction, allergic: +. **Symptoms**: Pruritus. **Borders**: Irregular, slightly blurred, extending beyond the hapten contact area. **Structure**: Homogeneous all over the test area. **Morphology**: Erythema, edema, a few papules, and a tendency to form vesicles. **Evolution**: "Increasing severity" reaction

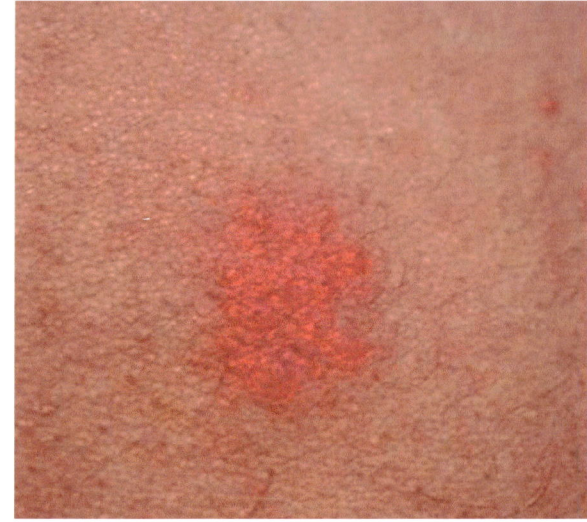

Fig. 7.69 Positive reaction, allergic: + + +. **Symptoms**: Pruritus. **Borders**: Irregular, blurred, extending well beyond the hapten contact area. **Structure**: Homogeneous all over the test area. **Morphology**: Erythema, edema, a few papules, very evident vesicles, sometimes confluent forming blisters. **Evolution**: "Increasing severity" reaction

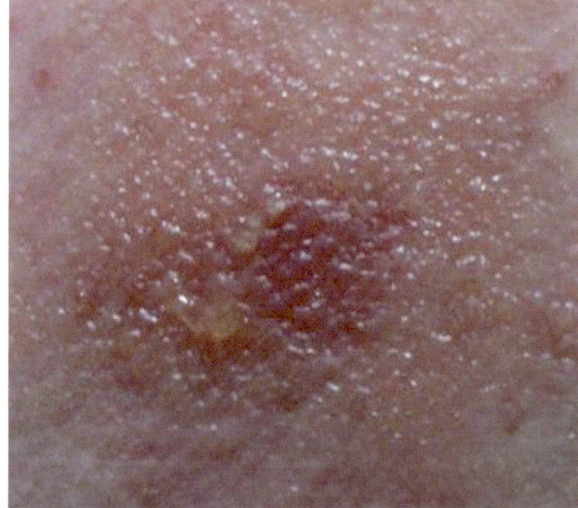

Suggested Reading

Barbaud A, Gonçalo M, Bruynzeel D et al (2001) Guidelines for performing skin tests with drugs in the investigation of cutaneous adverse drug reactions. Contact Dermatitis 45:321
Bruynzeel DP, Ferguson J, Andersen K et al (2004) Photopatch testing: a consensus methodology for Europe. J Eur Acad Dermatol Venereol 18:679
Bruze M, Svedman C (2015) Patch testing. In: Johansen JD, Thyssen J, Lepoittevin J-P (eds) Quick guide to contact dermatitis. Springer, Berlin
Bruze M, Condé-Salazar L, Goossens A et al (1999) Thoughts on sensitizers in a standard patch test series. The European Society of Contact Dermatitis. Contact Dermatitis 41:241
Bruze M, Isaksson M, Gruvberger B et al (2007) Recommendation of appropriate amounts of petrolatum preparation to be applied at patch testing. Contact Dermatitis 56:281
Cronin E (1972) Clinical prediction of patch test results. Trans St Johns Hosp Dermatol Soc 58:153
De Groot A (2008) Patch testing. Test concentrations and vehicles for 4350 chemicals. Acdegroot Publishing, Wapserveen
de Ward-van der Spek FB, Darsow U, Mortz CG et al (2015) EAACI position paper for practical patch testing in allergic contact dermatitis in children. Pediatr Allergy Immunol 26:598
Fonacier L, Noor I (2018) Contact dermatitis and patch testing for the allergist. Ann Allergy Asthma Immunol 120:592
Frosch PJ, Geier J, Uter W et al (2011) Patch testing with the patients' own products. In: Johansen JD, Frosch PJ, Lepoittevin J-P (eds) Contact dermatitis. Springer, Berlin
Gonçalo M, Ferguson J, Bonevalle A (2013) Photopatch testing: recommendations for a European photopatch test baseline series. Contact Dermatitis 68:239
Goossens A (2009) Alternatives aux patch tests. Ann Dermatol Venereol 136:623
Johansen JD, Frosch PJ, Lepoittevin J-P (eds) (2011) Contact dermatitis. Springer, Berlin
Johansen JD, Aalto-Korte K, Agner T et al (2015) European Society of Contact Dermatitis guideline for diagnostic patch testing—recommendations on best practice. Contact Dermatitis 73:195
Johansen JD, Thyssen J, Lepoittevin J-P (eds) (2015) Quick guide to contact dermatitis. Springer, Berlin
Jonker MJ, Bruynzeel DP (2000) The outcome of an additional patch-test reading on days 6 or 7. Contact Dermatitis 42:330
Lachapelle J-M, Maibach HI (2009) Patch testing and prick testing—a practical guide. Springer, Berlin
Ramirez F, Chernobyl MM, Botto N (2017) A review of the impact of patch testing on quality of life in allergic contact dermatitis. J Am Acad Dermatol 76:1000
Rietschel R, Fowler JF (2010) Fisher's contact dermatitis. BC Dekker, Lewiston, ME
Rustemeyer T, Elster P, John SM et al (eds) (2012) Kanerva's occupational dermatology. Springer, Heidelberg
Yu J, Atwater AR, Brod B et al (2018) Pediatric baseline patch test series: Pediatric Contact Dermatitis Workgroup. Dermatitis 29:206

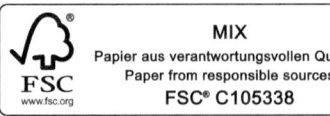

If you have any concerns about our products,
you can contact us on
ProductSafety@springernature.com

In case Publisher is established outside the EU,
the EU authorized representative is:
**Springer Nature Customer Service Center GmbH
Europaplatz 3, 69115 Heidelberg, Germany**

Printed by Libri Plureos GmbH
in Hamburg, Germany